Pelican Books
You and Your Heart

Paul Kezdi is Director of the Cox Research Institute and
Associate Dean for research and Professor of Medicine at
Wright State University School of Medicine.

Paul Kezdi

You and Your Heart

How to Take Care of Your Heart for a Long and Healthy Life

PENGUIN BOOKS

Penguin Books Ltd, Harmondsworth, Middlesex, England
Penguin Books, 625 Madison Avenue, New York, New York 10022, U.S.A.
Penguin Books Australia Ltd, Ringwood, Victoria, Australia
Penguin Books Canada Ltd, 2801 John Street, Markham,
Ontario, Canada L3R 1B4
Penguin Books (N.Z.) Ltd, 182–190 Wairau Road, Auckland 10,
New Zealand

First published in the U.S.A. 1977
Revised edition first published in Great Britain
by Proteus (Publishing) Ltd 1979
Published with further revisions in Pelican Books 1981

Made and printed in Great Britain by
Richard Clay (The Chaucer Press) Ltd, Bungay, Suffolk
Set in Monotype Baskerville

Contents

Preface   7

Introduction: The Great Killer   9

PART ONE: WHAT YOU SHOULD KNOW ABOUT YOUR HEART

1. How Your Heart Works   19
2. The Causes of Heart Disease   33
3. The Symptoms of Heart Disease – True and False   61
4. Treatment and Research   74

PART TWO: THE FACTORS THAT AFFECT YOUR HEART

5. Your Sex and Your Heart   83
6. Your Heredity and Your Heart   87
7. Your Age and Your Heart   91
8. Your Physique and Your Heart   94
9. Your Emotions and Your Heart   98
10. Your Environment and Your Heart   102
11. Your Work and Your Heart   106
12. Your Food and Your Heart   110
13. Your Drink and Your Heart   116
14. Your Sleep and Your Heart   120
15. Your Sex Life and Your Heart   122

16. Smoking and Your Heart   125
17. Exercise and Your Heart   135

PART THREE: HOW TO KEEP YOUR
              HEART HEALTHY

18. How to Choose Your 'Heart-Saver'
    Food and Drink   143
19. How to Stop Smoking   151
20. How to Plan and Perform an Exercise
    Programme   162
21. How to Relax   175
22. How to Live Enjoyably after a Heart
    Attack   185

    Endpiece   189
    Glossary   191
    Appendix I   199
    Appendix II   205
    Index   209

Preface

Dr Paul Kezdi has written this book in an attempt to bridge the gap between the lay reader with an intelligent interest in his heart and the specialized medical knowledge about the heart and its function, how it is deranged in disease, and what modern cardiologists feel one should do about it.

He is well qualified to do so, for not only is he a distinguished scientist, the Director of the Cox Research Institute, who has made a distinguished reputation particularly for his contributions to our knowledge of how blood pressure is controlled in subjects with high blood pressure, but he is also a practising physician in a busy modern hospital.

This is a sensible and well-balanced book. It is not a prejudiced or one-sided account of the evils of bad diet, but takes a broader view and particularly concentrates on some of the positive things that one can do to develop a healthy circulation.

Health education of this sort is an evolutionary rather than a revolutionary process. Results take time to appear. In the United Kingdom we have often overtly or covertly poked fun at the American obsession with health during the last decade. However, the recent trends in mortality from vascular diseases in the United States suggest that this campaign is at last beginning to bite and there appears to be a reduction in these diseases. It is noteworthy that during the last year or two some of this effort has begun to influence people on this side of the Atlantic as well. More people are taking exercise, there is a switch either from smoking to non-smoking, or from smoking cigarettes to pipe or cigars.

Although there is a good deal of controversy about diet there is no doubt that our national eating habits have changed profoundly in the last 25 years, and we do take much more of our diet as fat compared with carbohydrate than formerly. This book reviews some of the evidence concerning the role of fat in coronary disease. It also points out the importance of high blood pressure and other factors such as smoking history, sex and family history in the overall causation of vascular disease.

It is not an alarmist book and it could be well recommended to young and middle-aged alike. It deserves to succeed and I think it will.

Peter Sleight, M.D., D.M., F.R.C.P.
Radcliffe Infirmary, Oxford

Introduction

THE GREAT KILLER

Why take care of your heart?

There are some good reasons.

Heart disease is the most frequent cause of death and disability in the Western world including the United Kingdom.

Hundreds of thousands of heart attacks occur each year in Britain alone and almost one half of the victims die during the first attack. The death from heart and vascular disease accounts for approximately one half of all fatalities, including those caused by cancer, accidents, and other diseases. To say it in another way, heart disease causes at least as many deaths as all the other major killers put together.

Even more alarming than these chilling statistics is the estimate that millions of Britons now have some form of heart or blood vessel disease. Of these diseases, high blood pressure is the most prevalent. Next comes coronary heart disease. This includes people who have either had a heart attack or have a history of chest pain with confirming diagnostic signs of heart disease.

As great a tragedy of these diseases themselves is the fact that many of the people afflicted are unaware of their danger. And it has to be recognized that unknowingly you may be among this group, and are unaware of the fact only because the condition has not yet reached the symptomatic stage.

In the light of the figures from the Western world, including Britain, it is impossible to doubt that we have a major epidemic on our hands. The disease is as crippling and costly as any in our history. Yet, how many of us feel horrified enough to do something about it? It seems that the large number of individuals without symptoms dramatic enough to tell them that they have the beginnings of heart disease are able continually to lull themselves into a false sense of security. In most cases, only a major catastrophe, such as a heart attack or a stroke, makes them and their loved ones totally – and painfully – aware of their problem.

The resulting physical, mental, and economic suffering of individuals and families is so enormous that it cannot be expressed in money or in any other measurable element. Truly there is no one who does not have a relative or friend who has not already been stricken by this modern 'plague', or will not be in the near future.

How is it that this apathy can continue when we consider that simple guidelines for effective preventive action are available to everyone. These are, as we shall see later, becoming better and better known to the public almost by the day.

The answers to these questions are not easy. It is perhaps an oversimplification to say that people tend not to take preventive action, or even to acknowledge the existence of a problem or danger, until it strikes them personally. Yet, as we noted, almost nobody is unacquainted with heart disease. What, then, is the matter with us? Is it that we intentionally close our eyes to what we may think is inevitable, like death itself? Are we simply too fatalistic in our thinking about our own health and well-being? Are we too busy to care? Or could it be that we are simply too lazy? Or too uninterested?

All the evidence suggests that none of these factors is really the answer. We do care about things affecting our well-being, our country, the quality of our lives, our communities, our homes, our children, our schools, and so on. Indeed, the Western world has progressed scientifically, technically, and culturally beyond imagination. We are concerned about progress, order, cleanliness, efficiency, health, and social well-being.

We have developed labour-saving gadgets and machines, industrial and environmental preventive programmes, and so on. Our labour-saving machines promise trouble-free operation for many years provided we follow the instructions for preventive maintenance. Thus, the first thing we do when we buy a piece of equipment – a washing machine, a lawn mower, a power saw – is to read and study the operating and preventive maintenance instructions. We want to know where all the bits and pieces are, how to set the controls for smooth operation, how to replace parts, how to fuel and lubricate, and so on. We do this to be able to take care of at least simpler maintenance ourselves, to ensure extended trouble-free function, because we like to know how to do things and because we have paid hard-earned money for these prized possessions.

Is our heart not much more precious to us than these gadgets and machines?

If the answer is yes – and I cannot imagine anyone answering no – how is it, then, that many of us know and care so very little, if anything, about the most amazing machine we possess, our own heart?

The blindness of the individual to the risk of heart disease is even more puzzling when compared to reactions to other diseases. For example, how would you feel and what would you do if you suspected that you had been infected with leprosy? Like heart disease, this infectious disease also often lies dormant without making its victims obviously ill for ten or more years. It is a certainty that in this situation you would be horrified, and rush to seek every medical help available, even without having experienced the slightest symptom or ill effect. But you know, of course, that leprosy is a disease of the tropics, and that it is under control in most parts of the world. Consequently, the thought of contracting it never occurs to you, and you would not fear this illness even if it did. Yet the plain fact is that hardening of the arteries and high blood pressure do threaten you, even though you may have no signs or thoughts of them whatsoever.

The proof lies in the effect of these and other heart and circulatory diseases on the life expectancy of people. Statistics indicate that life expectancy of people in the Western world, after the age of 40, has changed very little since the turn of the century. The major increase in life expectancy occurred mostly in babies and young individuals, as the result of great reductions in infant deaths and deaths from infectious diseases. Deaths from heart disease (and probably from cancer) after the age of 40 have actually increased since 1900.

Thus, to be totally realistic, any young man or woman of 30 to 50 today has only slightly better a chance than in 1900 to live a productive life into ripe old age. And the single greatest reason why not is heart and circulatory disease, born of ignorance and apathy about both the diseases themselves and the life-style factors that cause them.

A perspective of these factors is contained in statistics on the incidence of coronary heart disease in countries of other than Western culture and life style. For example, the incidence of coronary heart disease in Japan is 15 to 30 per 10,000 population per year, while in the United Kingdom it reached approximately 140 per 10,000, and the United States is 177 per 10,000 population per year. The incidence is close to ten times higher. Other countries, such as Greece, Yugoslavia, and Italy, fall between these two figures, while Finland, with 198 per 10,000 population per year, exceeds even the United States.

We shall show later that atherosclerosis is the cause of coronary heart disease. One of the primary culprits in the development of atherosclerosis is high blood cholesterol, which in turn is directly related to the amount of saturated fat you ingest in your food. It thus becomes revealing to see the statistics regarding saturated and unsaturated fat intake as a percentage of daily calorie intake in different countries. The lowest intake in saturated fats has been shown to exist in certain communities of Japan, and the highest in Finland. The United States and Holland follow closely while Great

Projected life expectancy of men in the U.K.

AGE	LIFE EXPECTANCY (YEARS)				
	1931	1951	1961	1971	1974
0	58.4	66.2	67.9	68.6	69.3
1	62.1	67.5	68.6	69.1	69.3
30	38.1	40.2	40.9	41.2	41.7
45	25.5	26.4	26.9	27.2	27.6
60	14.4	14.7	15.0	15.1	15.6

Source: Social Trends, no. 8, 1977, Government Statistical Service, HMSO, 1977

MEN 40–59, CHD-FREE AT ENTRY
CHD INCIDENCE/10,000/YEAR

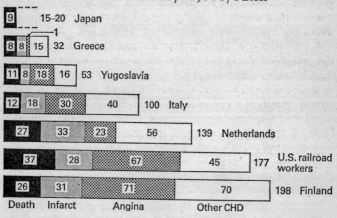

Death   Infarct   Angina   Other CHD

Age-standardized average yearly CHD incidence rates per 10,000 of 12,529 men aged 40–59, judged to be free of CHD at the outset, followed for five years. Non-fatal CHD incidence in Japan is not precisely indicated because the relevant five-year clinical and ECG records were not independently reviewed at the University of Minnesota centre.

Source: Ancel Keys, 'Coronary Heart Disease in Seven Countries', Circulation, 41, Supplement I, 1970. Used by permission of the author and the American Heart Association, Inc.

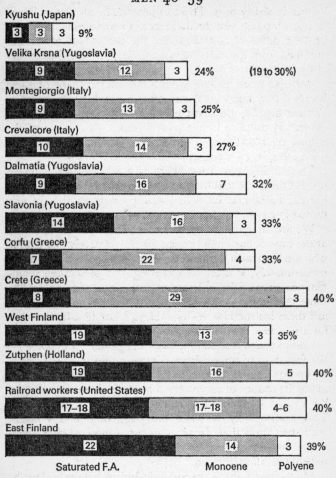

AVERAGE % CALORIES FROM FATS
MEN 40–59

Kyushu (Japan)
3 | 3 | 3 | 9%

Velika Krsna (Yugoslavia)
9 | 12 | 3 | 24% (19 to 30%)

Montegiorgio (Italy)
9 | 13 | 3 | 25%

Crevalcore (Italy)
10 | 14 | 3 | 27%

Dalmatia (Yugoslavia)
9 | 16 | 7 | 32%

Slavonia (Yugoslavia)
14 | 16 | 3 | 33%

Corfu (Greece)
7 | 22 | 4 | 33%

Crete (Greece)
8 | 29 | 3 | 40%

West Finland
19 | 13 | 3 | 35%

Zutphen (Holland)
19 | 16 | 5 | 40%

Railroad workers (United States)
17–18 | 17–18 | 4–6 | 40%

East Finland
22 | 14 | 3 | 39%

Saturated F.A.   Monoene   Polyene

Average percentage of dietary calories provided by saturated, monoun, and polyunsaturated fatty acids.

Source: Ancel Keys, 'Coronary Heart Disease in Seven Countries', *Circulation*, 41, Supplement I, 1970. Used by permission of the author and the American Heart Association, Inc.

Britain is closely next. There appears to be an almost linear relationship between the incidence of coronary heart disease in these different countries and the percentage of calories obtained from saturated or animal fats. We shall be elaborating on this later.

Perhaps more people would take better care of their hearts if they knew what an amazing machine the heart is.

Your heart is the most efficient machine that has ever existed. It contains in one both a pump with valves to distribute the blood flow in the desired direction, and a motor generating its own energy to activate the pump.

The efficiency of your heart as a self-propelling pump several times exceeds that of any man-made engine, and its normal functional life when healthy outlasts that of any humanly created technological marvel.

We are all endowed by nature with this perfect machine at the time of our birth (except for the relatively few people who are born with defective hearts). What we are not given, unfortunately, is a set of operating and preventive maintenance instructions, at least not in the form of a booklet like those that come with a new dishwasher or hairdryer. But are these instructions really missing? Let us consider that for a moment.

Comparative studies of animal behavioural physiology – the functions of physical life – have taught us that there is no known animal species that would intentionally harm itself or its chance of survival. All animals protect themselves by instinct from weather, enemies, adverse environments. They instinctively eat foods that fulfil their bodily needs. And they train their faculties to the utmost to give themselves the best chance to complete the full life span that nature has allotted them.

Man, essentially, is an animal, and in his early days he shared those characteristics with all other occupants of the planet. But that was long ago. Today, of all the species of the earth, man is the only one that repeatedly fails to make proper use of his instincts. And this situation is worsening in the Western world, despite all the powerful and ever-increasing efforts of medical science in recent years to make man aware of the fact that preventive maintenance of his body, and especially of his heart, is the only way to assure a long and healthy life. And all this despite the fact that the basic rules of preventive health care are often no more than simple common sense.

This book tells you how to apply your common sense and your instincts to the preventive maintenance of your heart. It is not intended to create fear, nor to take away the joy of living by recommending onerous, cumbersome, or expensive regimens. Its purpose is simply to help you as easily as possible to lessen the risk of suffering a fatal or disabling heart attack.

No one wants to be told by his doctor that his life-sustaining pump is failing and that no maintenance can now restore its function. After all, replacement techniques (transplants, artificial hearts, etc.) are still very far from being both effective and within the reach of the average man.

If you are reading this book, you will most likely admit to yourself that you have at some time been in fear of heart disease, especially if you are a middle-aged male. There is no need to live with such fear any longer. All you have to do is learn how to care for your heart, then do it. And you will be surprised at what little effort that takes, once you have formed the habit.

PART ONE

What You Should Know
About Your Heart

How Your Heart Works

There is much that you can do to preserve your heart. But first it will help you to know how it works.

We have said that the heart is a pump – but *what* a pump! Your heart begins its unceasing work before your birth, and, if you are healthy and lucky, it will pump uninterruptedly for 80 to 90 years or more. If for any reason it should stop pumping for more than four minutes, you would die.

When you are resting, your heart pumps 10 pints (approximately 5 litres) of blood each minute (called 'cardiac output'). It can increase its pumping up to five times this amount, or to $6\frac{1}{4}$ gallons (25 litres) per minute during heavy exercise for brief periods of time. It pumps on the average 3,000 to 5,000 gallons of blood every twenty-four hours; or 1,400,000 gallons every year; or 100 million gallons during a lifetime of 80 years – enough to fill the tanks of 2,100 four-engined Boeing 747 airliners.

Your heart does this monumental amount of work by ejecting 2 to 3 ounces of blood with each contraction or beat (called stroke volume), when pumping 60 to 70 times each minute during rest; and up to 4 to 5 ounces per beat while contracting at a maximum of 180 to 190 beats per minute (maximum heart rate) during heavy exercise, as in the case of the highly trained athlete. The maximum pumping capacity (maximum cardiac output) of the heart varies from individual to individual, but generally the average healthy person's maximum capacity is approximately two-thirds that of the trained athlete.

The basic purposes of the pumping function of your heart

are to supply the life-giving oxygen, nutrients, minerals, and water needed by the cells of all your organs, and at the same time to remove from them metabolic by-products, excess water, and carbon dioxide. The blood kept in constant motion by your heart also circulates important regulatory substances, called hormones, throughout your body.

Your blood reaches your organs initially through a branching vascular tree which eventually ends at the microscopically tiny blood vessels, the capillaries. The capillaries number in the billions, and across their walls your blood 'feeds' the trillions of cells that make up your body.

Should all your blood vessels be joined end to end, instead of running in parallel, they would reach almost $2\frac{1}{2}$ times around the earth at its equator – some 60,000 miles. The pumping force of your heart moves your blood through this tremendous network of vessels and back to your heart in approximately 10 seconds.

Even more amazing than these fundamental mechanics of life are the intricate regulatory functions governing the heart and blood vessel system that enable it to adapt to the ever-changing needs of your body. Your blood does not flow at a constant rate through all your organs, but adapts momentarily to the specific needs of each particular organ, depending on the conditions existing in each organ at any given moment. For instance, when you perform a jogging exercise, the blood flow to your leg muscles quickly increases through dilation of the blood vessels in your legs in order to meet the demand of the leg muscles, while the flow to other less active areas, such as the gut, decreases through constriction of the blood vessels in that area. Comparably, when you rest after a large meal your gut receives a proportionately larger flow of blood, and, when you concentrate and study, your brain receives a proportionately larger flow.

These fine adjustments of blood flow are necessary because, if all the blood vessels were to dilate at the same time, the heart would have to pump 90 pints of blood per minute,

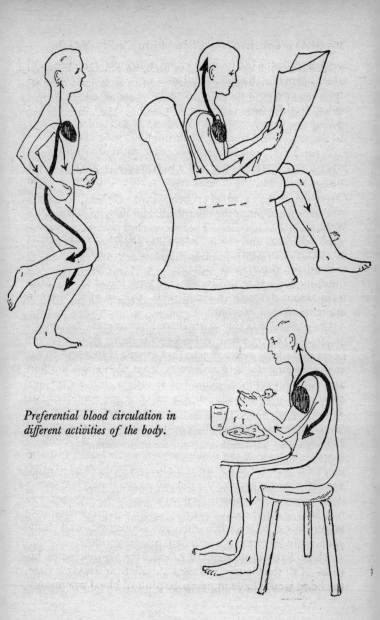

Preferential blood circulation in different activities of the body.

which it cannot do (as we have seen, 50 pints per minute is the heart's maximum capacity even in a trained athlete). The result would be that the blood pressure would drop to zero, and the individual would bleed to death into his own blood vessels.

HEART CHAMBERS AND HEART VALVES

Your heart has four chambers. Two of them, known as ventricles, are pumping chambers, and two, known as atria, are collecting chambers. There is one left pumping chamber (left ventricle) and one left collecting chamber (left atrium), and also one right pumping chamber and one right collecting chamber (right ventricle and atrium). The two ventricles are divided by a partly muscular and partly membranous wall, called the septum, and the atria are divided by a mostly membranous dividing wall. These dividing walls are non-porous, and do not allow communication or exchange of blood between the ventricles or atria.

Each atrium communicates with the ventricle of its own side (right atrium with right ventricle and left atrium with left ventricle), but is separated by a valve which is open part of the time and closed part of the time within the cycle of one heart beat. These valves consist of fine membrane tissue, and they are attached to the wall at the dividing line between the ventricle and the atrium around the inner surface of the heart.

The free ends of the valves are attached at several points to fine strings of tissue, which are anchored to protruding muscle bundles, called papillary muscles, in the ventricle. These leaflet-like tissue valves function like the sails of a yacht, ballooning when the pressure increases in the ventricle just as a sail balloons under the force of the wind. The touching of their free ends when the valves balloon causes them to fit tightly, closing off communication between the ventricle and the atrium. When the pressure in the ventricle drops, the valve leaflets collapse, just as the sail collapses when the wind ceases, which opens up communication and allows entrance of blood from the atrium into the ventricle.

Two other valves, somewhat different in nature, are

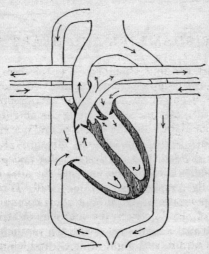

Schematic diagram of the heart and circulatory system. The heart receives the 'tired' blood (venous) from the lower and upper part of the body by the right atrium (your left) and ejects it by the right ventricle into the pulmonary vascular system. After oxygenation the blood returns to the left atrium (on your right) and is ejected by the left ventricle through the aorta to the head and lower part of the body.

situated at the exits of the two pumping chambers, where they communicate with two large blood vessels into which they pump their contents. The purpose of these valves is to prevent a backflow of blood into the pumping chamber when the chamber relaxes after each contraction.

Thus, the two different types of valves connected to each of the heart chambers alternately close and open. The valve at the entrance of the pumping chamber opens during its relaxation, and the valve at the exit opens during contraction of the pumping chamber. Each valve closes during the opposite condition of the ventricles. In this way, pumping of blood in one direction only is assured.

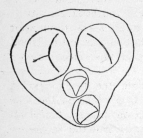 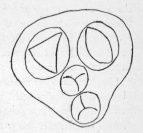

Schematic cross-sectional diagrams of the four heart valves. The left diagram shows the aortic and pulmonary valves (upper two) closed, the valves between the left atrium and ventricle (on your lower left) and the right atrium and ventricle (lower right of the left diagram) open. The diagram on your right shows the opposite condition.

We have said that the heart has two receiving and two pumping chambers communicating with each other. As the blood returns through the veins into the right atrium, after it has performed its task of perfusing and nourishing your organs, it flows over to the right ventricle when the valve is open. From there it is pumped into a large blood vessel called the pulmonary artery. This big artery directs the blood into the branching arteries of the lung, from which the arteries again divide into very small blood vessels in the walls of the small air sacs of the lung, where the exchange of oxygen inhaled by the lung and carbon dioxide released by the blood takes place.

Carbon dioxide, which is the metabolic product of cellular breathing, is released by the haemoglobin of the red blood cells, which carry it to the air sacs (alveoli). As you breathe, the carbon dioxide is exchanged for the oxygen concentrated in your air sacs. The oxygen finds its way through the walls of the air sacs and small blood vessels to replace the carbon dioxide delivered by the haemoglobin. The oxygen-rich blood is then collected again into larger blood vessels, which eventually enter the left receiving chamber (atrium) and then the left pumping chamber of the heart through the valvular action we have described. From here, the blood is pumped into the aorta, the largest blood vessel of your body. The aorta then carries the blood to the different organs according to their need, as we described earlier.

Owing to a remarkable precision, the two pumping chambers keep exactly in step with each other, neither one outdoing the other (should they get out of step, the blood would eventually be pumped in larger amounts to one or other side of the system). This phenomenal precision of the pumping mechanism is vitally important to life in that it regulates the amount of blood pumped per unit of time, which is called cardiac output. Cardiac output can vary between 8 to 12 pints per minute at rest, and up to 50 pints during heavy exercise, without disturbing the balance between the two sides of the heart.

YOUR HEART'S OWN BATTERY AND NERVOUS SYSTEM

How is such remarkable precision possible?

It is accomplished by your heart's own nerve centre, which regulates heart beat and muscle contraction and synchronizes the pumping action of the two ventricles with the contraction and relaxation of the two atria.

The nerve centre of this overall precision mechanism is in your heart itself. It is a tiny little 'battery', called the sinus node, in the wall of the right atrium, composed of special muscle and nerve cells that are charged by chemical mechanisms. The sinus node functions as an electric capacitor, which generates an electrical current as it periodically discharges at a given potential difference. This current is conducted through nerve bundles first to the muscles of the atria, then to the ventricles. The electrical discharge and conduction is extremely precise, and, by occurring at exact time intervals, it causes the heart muscles

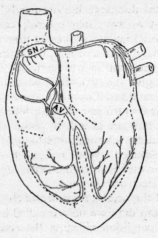

The sinus node (heart's 'battery') and conduction system as shown diagrammatically. S N = sinus node; A V = atrioventricular node. Both extend to the conduction system. See text.

to contract in just the exact sequence necessary to pump the blood.

The periodic discharge of this little battery coincides with what you recognize as your heartbeat. The rate of the heartbeat in any individual can vary between 60 and 90 at rest, and 140 and 190 maximum during heavy exercise.

While the mechanism of the heart's battery is automatic, its actual rate of discharge is constantly modified by messages coming from the central nervous system, the brain. The brain knows when the rate of discharge, or heart rate, should be increased and when it should be decreased. The little battery follows your brain's command to determine your heart rate at any given time.

The nerve bundles conducting the impulses from the sinus node to the heart muscles also possess a very remarkable mechanism. These nerves first branch within the muscles of the atria, making them contract simultaneously immediately after an electrical discharge has occurred. The impulse is then delayed in a 'switching centre', called the atrio-ventricular (or AV) node, by an exact time period, namely 120 to 200 thousandths of a second, before being forwarded to and causing the ventricles to contract. The purpose of this delay is to give the atria time to contract while the ventricles are relaxed and the valves between them are open. This ensures that the atria and the ventricles never get out of sequence – that they are exactly in phase with each other.

The spread of the electrical discharge throughout the heart muscle, projected to your body surface and recorded from metal plates attached to your arms, legs, and chest, is, of course, your electrocardiogram.

Disruption of the precise sequence of the spread of electrical current from the sinus node is called heart block, and is caused by a condition affecting the conduction of the electrical current from the atria to the ventricles. Heart block is a serious problem, in that it disturbs the synchronization of the contraction of the atria and the ventricles so that the ventricles contract independently at a very slow rate.

Heart block can be corrected by implanting in the heart an artificial electrical pacemaker, which stimulates the ventricles to contract by replacing the heart's own electrical impulse, thereby restoring the proper rate and sequence of pumping.

YOUR HEART'S OWN BLOOD SUPPLY: THE CORONARY ARTERIES

In addition to supplying blood to the rest of your body, your heart also needs its own blood supply in order to generate its pumping force, and to trigger the automatic contraction of its muscles.

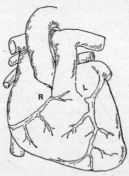

Front view of the heart showing branches of the left (L) and right (R) coronary arteries.

This blood supply is not derived from the flow of blood through your heart's chambers, but from your heart's own blood vessels, the coronary arteries. The coronary arteries are the first branches of the large blood vessel, the aorta, through which each contraction of your heart launches your blood on its journey around your body.

There are two coronary arteries, left and right, both of which divide into two major branches, then into ever more branches, and finally into small arteries and capillaries within the heart muscle, just like the arteries of all your other organs. The heart's blood is then collected and returned, through veins, into one large vessel called the coronary sinus, which enters the venous side of the heart, the right atrium. As we have seen, the right atrium is the collecting chamber of the heart for all 'used' blood returning from all your organs.

The blood flow to your heart, unlike the blood flow to your other organs, has a peculiarity in that it occurs mostly during the relaxation of the heart (called diastole), rather than during contraction (called systole). This is caused by the fact that, during maximum contraction, the pressure

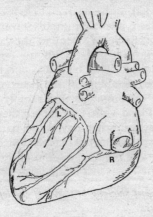

Back view of the heart showing distribution of the left (L) and right (R) coronary arteries towards the back wall of the heart.

within the heart muscle itself exceeds the pressure in the coronary arteries, which prevents free flow of blood for that brief period. For this reason, an important regulator of blood flow to the heart (known as coronary blood flow) is the pressure during the relaxation of the heart. This is expressed in the second number when your doctor measures your blood pressure, and is known as the diastolic pressure. The first number, or systolic pressure, indicates the peak pressure within your blood vessels when the heart contracts and ejects the blood.

If, for whatever reason, the blood pressure – and especially the diastolic pressure – is excessively low, the flow of blood to the heart can be impaired, resulting in lack of oxygen to 'feed' the heart. On the other hand, too high a diastolic pressure is just as harmful, in that it indicates increased resistance to the flow of blood throughout the blood vessels of the body, which results in an increased workload for the heart. High diastolic pressure is called hypertension, which is one of the main contributors to heart disease.

The flow of blood to the heart muscle is regulated by an intricate mechanism, involving impulses transmitted by the brain through the nervous system to the large and small coronary arteries, in concert with an equally intricate chemical mechanism. This chemical mechanism, called autoregulation, is the ability of the heart muscle itself to stimulate release of substances that rapidly and efficiently dilate the small blood vessels whenever they are suddenly called upon to deliver more oxygen to particular organs. When, for whatever reason, this chemical mechanism fails to trigger the delivery of required oxygen to the heart muscle, nerve endings signal that fact in the form of the heart pain commonly called angina.

THE CRITICAL MECHANICAL FACTORS

This, then, in very simple terms, is your heart. And what an amazing and marvellous life-giving mechanism it is!

What are the most important mechanical factors for its proper function in maintaining your blood circulation under the diverse activities of your daily life?

The first requirement is that your heart's miraculously efficient pumping action provides the necessary energy of contraction to meet the requirements of any given circumstance, which in turn depends on the adaptation of its own blood supply and nutrition to that given need. The second requirement is that the delicate regulation of your heart's function and its blood supply – as well as its regulation of blood circulation to your other organs – is optimally co-ordinated by your body.

If the blood supply, oxygen delivery, and delivery of nutrients to the heart muscle are impaired, the heart will fail to perform its pumping function properly, because its built-in motor, the heart muscle, is not receiving the necessary fuel. This is exactly what happens in one of the most common heart conditions, coronary heart disease.

Normally, all blood vessels, including the blood vessels to and within the heart itself, are lined with a beautifully smooth tissue called the endothelial lining, which has the property of preventing clotting or thickening of the blood within the vessel. Also, there are normally no bumps or narrow passages in the entire arterial tree, although the interior diameter of the vessels does, of course, decrease as they divide into smaller branches.

When bumps or narrow passages develop in different segments of the arterial tree – mostly in the larger arteries, including the coronary arteries – the condition known as atherosclerosis occurs, which will then result in gradual obstruction of blood flow through one or more vessels. The result is comparable to a water pipe becoming corroded with deposits of sludge or other debris. The interior diameter of the arteries at strategic points gradually narrows, usually over many years' duration. This process actually starts in childhood or early youth in people with high risk factors, and is completely without ill effects for decades in most individuals. However, as the years pass the risk factors increase in number until, with age, the process can become accelerated to the point of extreme danger.

For reasons not yet completely understood, blood vessels in certain organs are more likely to develop atherosclerosis than those in other organs. Among the blood vessels most frequently afflicted are those supplying the heart – the coronary arteries. Others, in decreasing order of risk, are the blood vessels of the brain, the legs, and the kidneys. We will go into more detail in later chapters about what is currently known about atherosclerosis, its mechanism, the factors predisposing an individual to its development, and particularly about how we can prevent the development of this insidious condition and its consequence, heart disease.

2

The Causes of Heart Disease

Your heart and your blood vessels are tied together as an inseparable system that supplies the life-giving blood to all your organs. As this system is inseparable, any illness, damage, or malfunction in any part of the system will affect the function of the entire system, and thereby impair to a greater or lesser degree the circulation of the blood as a whole. Yet the cardiovascular system has such a remarkable capacity to adjust and compensate that disturbances from malfunction of one or other part of the system are often tolerated by the afflicted person for a long time. It is indeed remarkable how long many individuals with relatively severe impairments can live a tolerable and functional life.

RHEUMATIC HEART DISEASE

We have seen that the majority of today's heart and vascular diseases are due to the insidiously slow development of atherosclerosis, and we will discuss later in detail what is known about the causes and mechanisms of this condition.

The second largest cause of heart disease is rheumatic fever, an affliction that is now known to be the result of an infection by bacteria that cause what is commonly known as strep throat. Not every throat infection is strep throat, but rather only the infection caused by the bacteria known as the beta haemolytic streptococcus.

Now, all of us in our childhood have had strep throat on occasion, because during winter the bacterial infection is easily spread among schoolchildren. Fortunately, only a few of us developed rheumatic fever from the infection, and only a certain percentage of those who had rheumatic fever suffered permanent damage to their heart.

Rheumatic fever is actually a second illness after the strep infection, and is thought to be the result of sensitizing the fine inner lining of the heart and vascular system, the endothelium, to the protein toxins of the bacteria. This causes a secondary inflammation of the inner lining, mostly around the heart valves, but sometimes in the small blood vessels of the heart muscle, and even of the outer lining of the heart itself. The healing of this inflammation often causes improper function of the valves through scarring and loss of elasticity. Once the toxin has sensitized the valves, repeated infections can produce new inflammation and progression of the scarring and malfunction.

Rheumatic fever usually develops when a streptococcus infection is uncontrolled for at least ten days, because it requires about that amount of time for sensitization to occur. Why some children and adults develop rheumatic fever and others do not has been the subject of study by many rheumatologists. Generally, it was found that a certain tendency to develop rheumatic fever can be inherited, but this is not a strong factor. Other studies seem to point to the fact that individuals living in poverty conditions, or who are undernourished to the point of receiving insufficient amounts of proteins, are most susceptible to rheumatic fever. Therefore, it is often a disease of the children of poverty areas, or persons undernourished for other reasons.

Sensitization to streptococcus toxins also has other manifestations, such as scarlet fever in children or adults, and kidney inflammation, or glomerulonephritis. Scarlet fever can also result in heart valve damage and chronic valvular disease affecting the blood circulation. Glomerulonephritis can result in chronic elevation of the blood pressure, and in this way impair the function of the heart, the circulation, and the kidneys. Rheumatic fever, scarlet fever, and glomerulonephritis can be placed in the same category, since the specific cause is the sensitization to the beta haemolytic streptococcus as a result of a strep throat infection.

We should stress that all of these secondary complications of the streptococcus infection, or strep throat, are much less frequent today than 20 or 30 years ago. The reason is that doctors learned that, if they could eradicate the infection *early* with the very effective antibiotics, particularly penicillin, no sensitization and secondary inflammation developed in the heart valves or the kidneys. For this reason, any throat infection with painful swallowing and elevated temperatures is suspect of strep infection, unless proved otherwise, and doctors normally take a swab and then probably treat it with antibiotics for some ten days because of the seriousness of the complications which may arise. This has led to a substantial decrease in the incidence of rheumatic fever following strep infections, so that rheumatic heart disease has become much rarer in the last 20 years than before the era of antibiotics.

Nevertheless, it is wise for parents always to call their family doctor when their children develop a painful throat infection with difficulty of swallowing, white patches on the tonsils, and fever. *Again, it is better to prevent the development of rheumatic fever than to try to find a cure after it has developed.*

CONGENITAL HEART DISEASE

When the heart or large blood vessels fail to develop normally before birth, a so-called congenital heart disease is present.

Approximately 16,000 children are born with congenital heart defects in the British Isles each year, and there are many causes and varieties of these defects, including some which can be transmitted by heredity and some which cannot.

In some cases, the heart defect is only one part of an overall congenital anomaly involving the central nervous system and other organs which may be caused by genetic abnormality. In other instances, some metabolic disorder of the mother during pregnancy – such as diabetes or hypothyroidism (low metabolism from low thyroid function) – is the cause of whatever heart malfunction is present. It has been shown in recent years in a number of cases that a relationship existed between heart defects and the mother's exposure in early pregnancy to infection such as German measles and other viruses, and more rarely to certain drugs. These viruses and drugs affected the development of the foetus at a critical time, causing an arrest of the development of specific parts of the heart and vascular system. Today some children with congenital heart disease, who have no other major organ malfunction, may undergo heart surgery that in many instances gives them the equivalent of a normal heart.

However, while heroic surgical procedures have often resulted in partial or almost total correction, sometimes of markedly malformed hearts and blood vessels, prevention is always the better course of action, even in congenital heart disease. Genetic counselling before marriage for those with genetic abnormalities should help to eliminate some of the malformations. Protection of pregnant mothers from virus diseases by immunization and isolation from specific virus-infected persons, especially in the most vulnerable stage of pregnancy, should prevent the development of some of the more frequent congenital heart malformations.

HEART MUSCLE DISEASE

Heart muscle disease can lead to acute and chronic heart failure, and may be caused by known or unknown factors. It is relatively rare in comparison to other heart diseases – the causes of which are fully known.

The condition can be caused by inflammation of the heart muscle, sometimes resulting from a general virus infection.

Fortunately, these acute heart muscle inflammations often heal without residual damage, but in some cases they may lead to chronic heart muscle weakness and heart failure. Since the heart muscle is the energy-producing and contracting element of the heart, any weakness in it must lead to some degree of inefficiency of the heart as a pump.

Among the known causes of chronic heart muscle weakness, the most important is chronic alcoholism. We have learned in recent years that alcohol, if taken regularly, even in relatively small amounts, can damage different organs of the body, particularly the central nervous system, the brain, the heart, the liver, and the kidneys. It has been shown that just one drink of two ounces of whisky will temporarily decrease the efficiency of the heart muscle. While the heart muscle easily recovers from this effect, repeated and frequent insults over a prolonged period may lead to chronic heart muscle weakness and heart failure.

Alcoholic heart muscle weakness (myocardiopathy) is seen quite frequently by every doctor. It is most prevalent not in the person who occasionally drinks large, intoxicating amounts, but rather in the people who regularly tolerate several drinks without showing signs of intoxication. Often, a combination of other conditions, such as existing valvular heart disease or infection, when combined with regular alcohol consumption, promotes the development of heart muscle disease.

In addition to these conditions, there are a number of other known causes of heart muscle weakness which are relatively rare, and are usually due to some form of metabolic disorder during the course of which heart muscle weakness may develop.

However, all of the above causes together are responsible for only a fraction of heart and vascular diseases in comparison with the two major problems facing particularly people of the Western civilized world: namely, high blood pressure (hypertension) and hardening of the arteries.

HIGH BLOOD PRESSURE
(HYPERTENSION) AND HEART DISEASE

We have shown earlier how very precisely your body regulates your blood pressure during the activities of your daily life.

A healthy heart can vary its pumping (cardiac output) five-fold between a resting state and heavy physical work with very little change in blood pressure. To explain this more precisely, in a healthy heart the average pressure – the mean between the systolic and diastolic pressure – does not change during exercise. What happens is that the systolic pressure increases due to the increased pumping force of the heart, while the diastolic blood pressure decreases due to dilatation of the blood vessels in the organs which have increased their activity – such as the leg muscles during jogging, for instance. The net result of the increased systolic pressure and the decreased diastolic pressure is that the average, or mean, pressure does not change significantly. In other words, the net result of the total *resistance* to blood flow in the blood vessel system is unchanged with a healthy heart, despite increases of the blood flow up to five times that of the resting cardiac output.

It has been recognized for quite some time that, in high blood pressure, the resistance to blood flow in the blood vessels is often increased. More recent studies have indicated that, in the early phases of hypertension, although the blood pressure may be normal at rest, during exercise there occurs an undue increase in both the systolic and diastolic pressure, thus causing an increase in the mean pressure. Researchers have further concluded that this is an early sign of the inability of the body to compensate for the increased blood flow during heavy physical activity.

When the blood pressure is elevated during rest, as it is in stable hypertension, the resistance in the blood vessels is more or less permanently raised. This permanent increase constitutes an increased workload for the heart, because now it has to work harder even during rest to maintain the blood flow necessary to perfuse all the organs of the body. And that, in simple terms, is why the heart may be damaged by the constant increase of its work that occurs in hypertension.

How does increased resistance in the blood vessels develop in certain individuals? What is the initial mechanism? What perpetuates the increased resistance? These questions have been the subject of very extensive investigations for many years, because high blood pressure is not only recognized as one of the major risk factors of coronary heart disease, but has also been found to promote hardening of the arteries (arteriosclerosis), leading to strokes, kidney disease, and the occlusion of arteries in extremities and other organs. In other words, high blood pressure is not only an increased strain on the heart, leading sometimes to heart failure, but also can be the cause of increased wear and tear on the blood vessels to the point where other illnesses are developed.

Since the regulation of the blood pressure in a normal healthy body is so precise, it is obvious that in high blood pressure something must have gone wrong with this regulation. Recognizing this fact, researchers have focused upon the constitution of the different factors involved in the regulation of the blood pressure. And, to make the story as short and simple as possible, these are the conclusions most of them agree upon today.

The calibre of the blood vessels (their resistance to blood flow) is modified by nerve impulses coming from the central nervous system, and also by blood-borne chemicals released from the adrenal glands, the kidneys, and maybe other glands. These mechanisms either constrict or dilate the blood vessels, depending upon the needs of the body. The nervous system and the kidneys receive information about the level of the blood pressure, and adjust their response according to the information supplied to them. In the simplest terms, when a decrease of blood pressure is registered, the nerve impulses decrease to allow the nervous system to increase its activity in order to constrict the blood vessels. Also at that time, the kidneys will send out their chemical constrictor to the blood vessels to raise the blood pressure.

While this mechanism is sufficient to adjust for rapid changes in blood pressure, there is another mechanism which provides for more prolonged changes by allowing the body to regulate the amount of water contained in the blood and tissues, which is called blood volume. This mechanism provides for the cyclic variations of seasonal conditions, and of the day and night, in order to maintain the blood pressure within normal range at all times.

Obviously, these are extremely delicate and vital mechanisms. The point to be made here is that, in high blood pressure, something has gone wrong with them.

It is now generally believed by researchers that, in approximately 15 per cent of all cases of high blood pressure, one or another identifiable defect in one of the regulatory mechanisms has initiated a chain of events leading to an alteration of the overall interrelated system of regulatory functions. However, in the majority of cases (85 per cent), the initiating factor is unknown. High blood pressure of this type is called primary hypertension (formerly, essential hypertension), indicating that the cause is unknown.

In cases where the initiating factor can be identified, present knowledge indicates it to be an interference with the blood flow to the kidneys. This condition exists when the artery to the kidney is narrowed, due either to an obstructing plaque from atherosclerosis or, more rarely, to excessive muscle tissue in the arterial wall, a rare congenital abnormality. Another cause of high blood pressure can be a tumour in the adrenal gland, producing excess blood-borne messengers which raise the blood pressure.

In the former cases, the obstructing plaque selectively decreases the pressure to the kidney, thereby falsely giving the impression to the kidney's sensory organs that the blood pressure in the entire body is decreased. The kidney then will produce more blood-borne messengers (renin) than needed, in order to raise the pressure within the kidney, which in turn leads to elevation of the blood pressure in the entire body. In the latter instances, the tumour in the adrenal gland will produce an excess amount of other blood-borne messengers (aldosterone) involved in blood-pressure regulation, again leading to elevation of the blood pressure.

It has been found that both of these mechanisms initially are opposed by other regulatory mechanisms of the body, such as the nervous system, but that these will soon be overcome by the overwhelming onslaught of the blood-pressure-raising, blood-borne messengers originating in the kidney or the adrenal gland. Eventually, the body's other regulatory mechanisms will adapt to, rather than oppose, the elevation of the blood pressure.

In both these cases, the condition, when properly diagnosed, can be cured by surgery, by repairing the arterial obstruction to the kidney, or by removing the adrenal tumour.

In the majority of cases of high blood pressure, however, we cannot detect any such overwhelming onslaught of blood-pressure-raising hormones or increased nerve impulses to the blood vessels. In these cases, the development of the increased blood pressure is slower, more insidious, and generally symptom-free, which is the reason why so many people in whom the condition exists do not know that they have high blood pressure.

What do we know about this primary hypertension? As I have said, we know very little about the initiating cause, although we know quite a bit about the mechanism of how the increased blood pressure is maintained. After the unknown initiating cause starts the chain of events, we can determine how the interrelated nervous system and hormonal or blood-borne messenger factors, originating in the kidneys and the adrenal glands, work in concert to constrict the small blood vessels and maintain the blood pressure at a high level all the time. And, deriving from the discovery of these different interrelated mechanisms, we now have several drugs which can act at different sites of the regulatory system to correct the malfunction at that site. That is why today we can so efficiently treat high blood pressure and prevent its complications.

There is some circumstantial evidence, mostly from the studies of the epidemiologists (researchers studying the frequency and relationship of disease to environmental and other factors in a population), that what starts the chain of events in high blood pressure may be related to hereditary factors within families and racial factors, to eating habits, and to nervous tension. What complicates the research is the difficulty of separating the family hereditary factors from life-style factors ingrained early in childhood in a family and usually carried throughout life. Nevertheless, identical-twin studies have indicated that heredity has a moderately strong influence on whether or not children will develop high blood pressure.

Racial factors seem to be indicated by the fact that blacks in the United States have a higher percentage of high blood pressure than whites. However, it is again difficult to separate inheritance from life-style factors, and the effects of social factors from those of hereditary. Blacks in Africa do not seem to have a high incidence of high blood pressure until involvement in the pressures of modern 'civilized' life changes their original life-style to that of the Western world. Thus, race would not seem to be a very important factor in the initiation of the abnormal mechanisms that lead to high blood pressure. The higher occurrence of high blood pressure among American blacks is probably mostly due to environmental and life-style factors.

What are these life-style factors?

Experimental studies have shown that excessive salt intake forced on rats can lead to high blood pressure (the rat being one of the animals most susceptible to high blood pressure). It has also been shown that Japanese fishermen living in the northern part of Japan, who use salt for food preservation, have a very high rate of high blood pressure. Studies in the United States have also indicated that individuals consuming large amounts of salt had a significantly higher rate of high blood pressure compared with those consuming moderate amounts of salt.

That there must also be other life-style factors would seem to be proved by the fact that individuals who are overweight have a higher rate of hypertension. Whether specific eating habits – or eating specific foods, excess protein, or specific proteins – have anything to do with high blood pressure is not known for sure, although these factors are occasionally suggested by some investigators but without adequate scientific basis.

Other causes have occasionally been suggested, such as drinking soft water, or ingesting excessive amounts of certain heavy metals, such as cadmium, through drinking water. Cadmium is present in lead pipes and may be dissolved by the water, especially when it is artificially softened, and it has been shown in research with animals that an excess amount of cadmium in drinking water can lead to kidney damage and thus to high blood pressure. But there is no existing evidence that heavy metals in the amount present in drinking water have a relationship to the cause of high blood pressure on a large scale in humans. Certainly, the Japanese fishermen in northern Japan do not have a plumbing system similar to ours, yet the number of hypertensives among them is much higher than in Britain or the United States.

How do the suspected initiating factors trigger the abnormalities in the blood-pressure-regulating mechanisms that lead to hypertension? It was suggested that heredity may be responsible for a tendency of the blood vessels to react excessively to normal nerve stimuli. This would result in an early thickening of the walls of the smaller vessels, which would in turn perpetuate the mechanism of abnormal regulation of blood pressure that is present in hypertension.

In early hypertension, however, the blood vessels' responsiveness is not increased; rather, the pumping force of the heart is increased, apparently an excessive response of the heart to nerve stimuli. What makes the heart pump excessively, even during rest, in the initial phase of high blood pressure is unknown. What is known is that increased retention of water and salt, by increasing the circulating volume of blood, can stimulate the heart to work excessively, causing elevated blood pressure through increased cardiac output. But, while water and salt (sodium) retention appears to be an early tendency in individuals with high blood pressure, this mechanism in itself is not sufficient to explain the increased cardiac activity. Nervous factors originating in the central nervous system, or in the heart itself, may be more responsible.

Researchers are continually studying this early phase of high blood pressure to try to learn something about the triggering mechanism, and are now quite excited about the possibilities provided by the development of a new strain of rats which develop high blood pressure spontaneously. This strain of rats was developed by New Zealand and Japanese investigators with special breeding techniques. In many ways, the mechanism of high blood pressure and its initial triggering mechanism after birth in these young rats seems to be quite similar to the mechanism known in human hypertensives. It is thus hoped that these studies will eventually shed light on the early triggering mechanisms leading to the vicious cycle of human hypertension.

However, irrespective of whatever this research might determine as the initial triggering mechanism, we can say today that high blood pressure can often be prevented by weight control or lowered by weight reduction. Overweight is an unsightly characteristic of a large number of people; and it is also unquestionably a promoter of hypertension.

Likewise, excessive salt intake cannot be good in that it

appears from most research to have at least *some* relationship to the development of high blood pressure. It is not known, however, whether or not excessive salt intake is the result of excessive salt appetite bred of the same mechanism that causes hypertension, or is a primary cause in itself.

Hypertension is popularly thought to be the result of increased mental tension and stress, and there is no doubt that psychologists who have studied this problem have detected certain similar personality characteristics in individuals with high blood-pressure. However, there is no convincing evidence that repressed hostility, overt ambition, and sheer 'drive' in and of themselves are responsible as initiators of hypertension. The best present evidence is that these are secondary characteristics, coincidental with hypertension. However, there is very little known about the role of the central nervous system, and of the complicated interrelationships the multiple regulatory mechanisms have with the central nervous system.

There are various possibilities as to where regulation can go wrong in the central nervous system, thereby affecting the entire body mechanism of blood pressure regulation. But there is still much to be done in this difficult area before we can definitely state whether or not the central nervous system, through nervous tension, psychological response to emotional stress, etc., is responsible as the primary factor for high blood pressure, or, indeed, whether it has any relationship to triggering the abnormal mechanism that leads to that condition.

What has to be faced, however, is that, *whatever* its causes, high blood pressure is an important risk factor in heart attacks, strokes, and other vascular diseases, and thus its prevention and treatment is a vitally important aspect of health care. Since some 5 million Britons and 22 million Americans have symptomatic or asymptomatic high blood pressure, the task appears to be overwhelming. Health agencies such as the British Heart Foundation, the American Heart Association and the National Heart and Lung

Institute are conducting extensive research and public education programmes for the detection, prevention, and treatment of the disease. Their chief hope for success is that individuals will take note of them, and then act accordingly in terms of life-style.

CORONARY HEART DISEASE

The predominant cause of coronary heart disease is hardening of the arteries, manifested by one or more obstructing plaques (called atherosclerosis) in the coronary arteries.

Atherosclerosis occurs when an obstructing plaque inhibits the blood flow to the heart muscle, particularly during increased work when the blood flow to the heart is increased to several times that of the resting flow. When this increase is inhibited by an obstructing plaque, the heart muscle does not receive the necessary oxygen in the area supplied by the blood vessel, and in consequence will not be able to perform the increased work demanded of it.

It has been shown that areas of the heart muscle suffering from oxygen lack do not contract, and sometimes even bulge in the opposite direction during the contraction (systole), when the pressure builds up in the heart chambers. Sensory nerve endings in the affected heart muscle are then irritated by the oxygen lack, and reflect the irritation to the chest wall in the form of pain or a sensation of 'heaviness'. This chest pain, when caused by oxygen lack in the heart muscle, is called angina pectoris. When it occurs during physical activity, it is called effort angina. Sometimes angina occurs even during rest or during very mild stimulation of the heart, such as in eating, or watching an exciting TV show, or during an animated discussion. In these instances, oxygen lack is already present during rest or little more than a resting state.

The coronary artery system normally has an unusually

large reserve. Chest pain is not experienced in usual daily activity before the inner calibre (the lumen) of an artery is obstructed more than 50 per cent.

Fortunately, nature has a remedial mechanism beyond even that point to correct decreased blood flow to a certain area of the heart muscle.

Although the branches of the large coronary arteries normally do not communicate with each other, they can develop such communication between an obstructed and a non-obstructed artery, the stimulus to the development of such communication being repeated and prolonged oxygen lack in the affected heart muscle. Development of this communication between obstructed and unobstructed blood vessels, called collateral circulation, takes place after weeks of obstruction in coronary heart disease. When such communications have developed, sometimes sufficient blood is shunted from the normal artery to the affected arterial system so that chest pain is reduced or disappears. However, this remedial mechanism is limited in itself, and also by the fact that the supplying blood vessel can also become obstructed. When this happens, chest pain reappears.

The obstruction of blood flow in a coronary artery reaches a critical point when the inner diameter of the blood vessel is decreased by 70 per cent or more. Then the smooth lining of the inner surface of the blood vessel, now also covering the obstructing plaque, can develop microscopically small tears, which can initiate clot formation in that area of the blood vessel. When this happens, an area of the heart muscle can lose its entire oxygen supply and, as a result, tissue dies in that area. Such massive injury to an area of the heart muscle is known medically as myocardial infarction, and is commonly called a 'heart attack'.

There is some indication that obstruction of blood flow to a coronary artery can occasionally be the result of a localized spasm of the wall of the artery. Such spasms occur mostly in areas opposite to already obstructing plaques, and rarely without the presence of such plaques. They can, however, reach such proportions that a myocardial infarction or heart attack develops.

The cause of such extreme localized spasms is unknown. It is suspected that they are due to localized nerve irritation in individuals having a tendency to excessive response of the vascular system to nerve stimuli. All the available evidence indicates, however, that vascular spasm of the coronary arteries is probably responsible for only a small fraction of the large number of heart attacks experienced in the Western world today.

In the great majority of cases, coronary heart disease and myocardial infarction are unquestionably the result of atherosclerosis. What is atherosclerosis, and what causes it? Unfortunately, there are no simple answers to these questions.

The obstructing atherosclerotic plaque seen in human arteries at autopsy, or during surgery for correction of arterial obstructions, is the end stage of a long process. The plaque bulging towards the inside of the blood vessel often has an irregular surface due to breaking and healing, resulting in scarring of the smooth layer of cells that normally line the surface of the blood vessel. The plaque itself consists of mushy, yellowish material collected in the vascular wall, sometimes containing hard calcium deposits which are the result of the healing process after rupture of the inner lining of the blood vessels that also cover the plaques. The plaque also destroys the normal tissues in the vascular wall.

Under a microscope, the plaques are seen to contain unusual yellowish, foamy-looking cells. The foamy material is composed of various types of fat particles which are inside special scavenger cells. Chemically, the plaques contain crystals which, upon analysis, are shown to be cholesterol. The plaques are surrounded by normal tissues which show inflammatory reaction and cell infiltration, such tissue reaction being a natural defence mechanism of the body to seal off and protect itself against any invasion by foreign materials. Atherosclerotic plaques can be localized in one place in the wall of an artery, but can also extend to the entire circumference of an artery, or to a whole segment of an artery.

The earliest sign of an atherosclerotic plaque is a barely visible yellowish streak on the inner surface of the artery, called a 'fatty streak', and it is a long process from here to the development of a full-blown, obstructing atherosclerotic plaque. Fatty streaks can sometimes be seen in childhood and youth as an early sign of atherosclerosis. In fact, post-mortem examinations of young American soldiers who died in the Korean war have shown that fatty streaks and early atherosclerotic plaques were present in 77 per cent, and 15 per cent had a narrowing of at least one coronary artery to 50 per cent of its original opening.

In other studies, an increased occurrence rate of fatty streaks has been found in post-mortem examinations of young victims of accidents in the U.S. as compared to Far Eastern and African natives. Nothing better indicates the high susceptibility of the Western population to athero-sclerosis.

To understand the mechanism of atherosclerosis, one has to understand first the metabolism of fats and cholesterol in the human body.

An important energy source for the function of the body, fats are chemically composed of a glycerine molecule bound to long-chain fatty acid molecules. Depending upon the number of free oxygen bonds in the fatty acid molecules (capable of forming bonds with iodine), the fats are either saturated, partly saturated, or unsaturated. Saturated fats have no free oxygen bonds because these are taken up by hydrogen atoms; they come mostly from animal products such as animal fat, meat, and butter. Unsaturated fats come from vegetable oils and some fish oils. Partially saturated fats come from both animal and vegetable products. The more a fat is saturated, the less liquid it is.

Fats are absorbed through the gut, and then travel in the

lymph vessels to the venous system as triglycerides. In the process they enter the blood circulation, which carries them to the liver. The liver has a central role in fat metabolism in that it converts fat either to a readily available energy source, or provides for the deposit of excess fat as an energy reserve in different bodily tissues. Thus, part of the liver's function is clearing the fats (triglycerides) from the blood circulation. Stored fats are then mobilized to provide energy as needed, but, when the source of energy is bountiful in the body these deposited fats are not utilized and any excess of them will lead to overweight.

Cholesterol, an important building stone for the body, is present in almost every cell. For example, bile salts are produced from cholesterol, and are very important in the digestion process. Cholesterol is also a very important chemical base with which the body produces the chemical messengers called hormones. Cholesterol therefore is obviously an important component of the human metabolism and is essential for life. But there is a problem with it, and the problem is that often we have too much of it.

The body receives cholesterol directly from certain foods, and can also produce its own cholesterol in the liver and other cells. Cholesterol travels in the bloodstream to the different target organs such as the adrenal gland, the pituitary, etc., where it is converted into different hormones (regulators of specific cell functions). The cholesterol level in the blood is, within certain variations, quite constant from day to day. This level is determined by the amount of cholesterol in the fats consumed – and particularly the amount of saturated fats ingested, in that these raise the level of cholesterol most significantly.

As cholesterol travels in the vascular system dissolved in the blood, it is exposed to the physical characteristics of the blood circulation. During its journey, some of the cholesterol filters across the fine inner lining of the blood vessel walls into the small lymph vessels which are present as a fine network in the walls of the arteries. Two factors particularly seem to be important in this mechanism: namely, the blood level of the cholesterol (its concentration in the blood), and the height of the blood pressure (pressure inside the artery). The higher the cholesterol concentration in the blood, the more cholesterol is filtered through the blood vessel walls. The higher the blood pressure, the more force (called filtration pressure) is exerted to move cholesterol across the wall.

When cholesterol level is low and blood pressure normal, the normal amount of cholesterol filtered through the arterial wall will easily pass to the lymph vessels. When cholesterol level is high and blood pressure (force of filtration) is increased, more cholesterol is filtered through the arterial wall. At some point, this increased amount of cholesterol will not be able to pass across the wall and will 'plug up' the 'filter' (the arterial wall) at certain points. In the initial phase, this process manifests itself as a 'fatty streak' in the arterial wall. Then, just as debris builds up in a blocked oil filter in your car, more cholesterol will be trapped as time goes on and the 'plug' will grow. Eventually, the cholesterol begins to act as a foreign material and produces an inflammatory reaction in the surrounding tissues, which in turn increases the size and changes the nature of the initial plug. Thus the atherosclerotic plaque is born.

Interestingly, the location of atherosclerotic plaques is predominantly around divisions and curvatures of the arterial system. This can be explained by the fact that arteries are exposed to the greatest force of the blood pressure (strain) around divisions and curvatures. Since filtration of cholesterol depends in part on the force of the blood pressure, atherosclerotic plaques are most predominant in the areas of greatest force acting on the arterial blood vessel system. A good parallel is the sludge and debris in a river collecting in areas of divisions and sharp curves.

You can immediately draw two conclusions from the above: (1) low concentration of cholesterol in the blood does not result in cholesterol entrapment in the arterial wall; (2) high blood pressure increases the force moving cholesterol across the arterial wall, which is why atherosclerosis is more prevalent in people with high blood pressure. Thus, elevated cholesterol and hypertension both promote the development of atherosclerosis. And their effect does not manifest itself as simple summation, but by multiplication.

We shall be looking more closely at cholesterol as a risk factor later on, but it is worth mentioning here that its level in an individual, after a specific diet containing known amounts of saturated fats, can actually be predicted. The level starts to change within a week of dietary change, and usually reaches a new plateau within three to four weeks, given no specific metabolic abnormality such as abnormal liver function, kidney disease, diabetes, etc.

There are other factors besides cholesterol in relation to blood pressure which influence development of atherosclerosis. Diabetes, low thyroid function (hypothyroidism), and certain kidney diseases promote the disease, since, by interfering with fat metabolism, these metabolic disorders act as risk factors by increasing cholesterol concentration in the blood. However, lowering the cholesterol level by correction of the metabolic disorder will decrease their risk effects.

Recent investigations indicate that there are perhaps differences in how the blood carries cholesterol and fats in different individuals. Fats and cholesterol are carried by proteins as lipoproteins, and, depending on the size of the protein molecule, the lipoprotein can be small or large. Small lipoproteins are called low-density lipoproteins, and large ones high-density lipoproteins. Very low-density lipoproteins have a greater tendency to increase cholesterol in the arterial wall, and thereby enhance the development of atherosclerosis. Some individuals may have a hereditary tendency to form these very low-density lipoproteins, and therefore atherosclerosis.

There is one other very strong risk factor, related to

smoking, the mechanism of which is not completely clear. When we talk about smoking as a risk factor, we usually refer to it as related to heart attacks. However, cigarette smoking as a risk factor probably has multiple roles.

First, it is a proven observation that heavy cigarette smokers usually have more extensive and earlier hardening of the arteries, and atherosclerotic plaques, than non-smokers, and this is true even when the heavy smokers have lower cholesterol levels than the individuals who have never smoked. Second, cigarette smoking has many other harmful effects on the body which could precipitate a heart attack in the presence of an obstructing plaque in a coronary artery. Cigarette smoking as a risk factor in heart disease must therefore be considered in two separate aspects.

Despite much research, it is still not clear how cigarette smoking promotes the development of atherosclerosis. Cigarette smoke contains nicotine, carbon monoxide, and other gases produced by the burning process, along with tar, other chemicals, and minute amounts of radioactive materials. Which of these substances is responsible for promoting atherosclerosis?

Studies of the effect of nicotine when inhaled in cigarette smoke have shown that it is a vasoactive drug, meaning that it acts on the smooth muscles of the vascular system to produce constriction of the small blood vessels, which slightly increases the blood pressure. At the same time, its effect on the heart is to increase heart rate. Smoking one or two cigarettes raises the blood pressure measurably and increases the heart rate in every individual, the effect lasting from 15 to 20 minutes and then subsiding. Can this blood-pressure-raising effect be responsible, when repeated sufficient times a day, for the promotion of atherosclerosis? It might seem so, in that we have seen that high blood pressure clearly increases the risk of developing atherosclerosis. However, the degree of blood-pressure increase deriving from cigarette smoking appears to be too small in and of itself to be responsible for the strong atherosclerotic risk factor of heavy cigarette smoking. Thus other effects must be considered along with this one.

One of these other effects could be the interference with the liver's clearing-factor mechanism that results from cigarette smoking. Nicotine has an adverse effect on the liver's ability to clear the increased blood fats, or triglycerides, after a meal, this function being delayed after smoking. However, there is no clear-cut evidence of a relationship between the level of triglycerides and coronary heart disease. Nor is there evidence that heavy cigarette smoking in and of itself raises the cholesterol level. Yet, even in the presence of only modestly increased blood cholesterol, cigarette smoking is a definite risk factor in atherosclerosis. What, then, is the mechanism of cigarette smoking in its so clearly demonstrable relationship to atherosclerosis?

Carbon monoxide is another ingredient in inhaled tobacco smoke, and it is present in considerably larger amounts than in the air of an average large town. Oxygen is bound in the lung to the haemoglobin molecule of the red cell, where it constitutes the important atom for the metabolic processes of the cells. Carbon monoxide also can bind with the haemoglobin molecule and, when the concentration of carbon monoxide is increased in the inhaled air, a contest develops between oxygen and carbon monoxide for binding with the haemoglobin. However, oxygen is handicapped in this battle, because haemoglobin has an affinity 250 times greater for carbon monoxide than for oxygen. So, even in the relatively low concentration inhaled with cigarette smoke, carbon monoxide will bind with a considerable number of haemoglobin molecules, thus preventing them from binding with oxygen. Carbon monoxide haemoglobin, being useless in the metabolic processes of the cells, thus interferes with cell breathing. Indeed, it has been shown that heavy cigarette smokers can have 10 to 15 per cent of their red blood cells bound by carbon monoxide, thus preventing those cells from performing their proper metabolic function.

Because of carbon monoxide's greater affinity to haemo-globin, its elimination from the red cell is also much slower – it takes, in fact, about two weeks after complete cessation of cigarette smoking for the body to eliminate carbon monoxide from the red cells. Since in a heavy cigarette smoker a con-siderable number of red cells cannot be used by the body in the breathing mechanism, there occurs an oxygen lack in the cells similar to that experienced when the concentra-tion of oxygen in the air is decreased at high altitudes. When that happens, the bone marrow is stimulated to compensate for the deficiency by increasing the number of the circu-lating red cells. And, indeed, heavy cigarette smokers have a statistically shown increase of their blood haemoglobin concentration and number of circulating red cells just like that occurring in people living at altitudes 10,000 to 14,000 feet above sea level. By increasing the thickness (viscosity) of the blood, this increase in cells has an effect on the ten-dency of the blood to clot. But there is as yet no clear-cut evidence that such increased red cell concentration has a relationship to the mechanism of the development of atherosclerotic plaques.

What has recently been discovered, however, is that heavy carbon monoxide concentrations in the blood in-crease the tendency of the inner lining of the blood vessels to filter cholesterol more easily. This occurs because the carbon monoxide affects the metabolism of the sensitive cells of the inner lining. And, of course, if in this way carbon monoxide enables cholesterol more readily to enter the blood vessel walls, it must be a factor in plaque formation.

This could explain how cigarette smoking promotes the development of an atherosclerotic plaque. Indeed, the mystery of the relationship between more severe and earlier atherosclerosis and heavy cigarette smoking, even in the absence of other risk factors, may soon be solved by the chronic carbon monoxide factor. The additional poisons in the cigarette smoke, such as tar and perhaps some radio-active materials, may promote lung cancer, but there is no evidence at present that they promote atherosclerosis. Of course, heavy cigarette smokers also have lung problems which can only aggravate the difficulty of oxygen exchange. When carbon monoxide is superimposed on this in the presence of an obstructing atherosclerotic plaque, the symptoms of breathlessness and chest pain, or angina pectoris, are increased.

Some consideration must now be given to the behavioural factors which might relate to coronary heart disease and myocardial infarction.

Much attention has recently been focused on the relationship of the psychological makeup of individuals to coronary heart disease and heart attack. Individuals have been classified from the standpoint of their psychodynamic behavioural characteristics into Type A and Type B. Type A individuals are said to be aggressive, impatient, time-conscious, superambitious men and women who have a significantly higher incidence of heart attacks than Type Bs, who are more placid and relaxed and less time-obsessed than their opposites.

In evaluating this classification as a risk factor, the same distinction has to be made as for cigarette smoking. The basic medical question is whether or not being a Type A is, in and of itself, an *independent* risk factor – the alternative possibility being that obstructive coronary atherosclerosis and Type A behaviour are the result of one or more other common factors.

The interesting point in this respect is that Mayer Friedman and Ray H. Rosenman, promoters of the concept that Type A behaviour is an independent risk factor, have themselves shown that *all* the other risk factors are more prevalent in Type A than in Type B people. For example, in Type A the average blood cholesterol is significantly higher, high blood pressure is more prevalent, and heavy cigarette smoking more frequent than in Type B. Could this be because the agressive Type As are more voracious eaters and drinkers, more tense and insecure, more in need of a crutch like smoking, because of their psychological makeup? If this is the case, then their increased atherosclerosis is perhaps caused *not* by their psychological makeup itself, but as a result of the *risk factors* it causes them to expose themselves to.

On the other hand, it could be that individuals who eat and drink more abundantly and smoke more heavily out of habit may develop aggressive Type A behavioural characteristics as a *result* of so doing. Type A behaviour would then be secondary to the overall life-style pattern which is associated more frequently with coronary heart disease.

In short, Friedman and Rosenman still owe us the proof that neither of the above is the case, but that Type A behaviour is, in and of itself, a *primary* mechanism.

Yet another factor that is influencing the coronary heart disease picture is physical activity, or rather the lack of it. Mechanized modern life has led to less and less energy expenditure by almost all classes of people. There is now convincing evidence that a steady high level of physical activity is a definite protective measure against heart attacks. It also appears that extended physical work, with periodic bouts of particularly heavy labour, is a more protective physical activity than the occasional once or twice a week on a tennis court, squash court, or jogging field. For example, in Evans County, Georgia, sharecroppers had less coronary heart disease and fewer heart attacks than their matched peers living a sedentary life in a nearby community. A more recent study, conducted on San Francisco Bay longshoremen, showed a seven-times higher death rate from heart attack in light-work category men than in heavy-work category men, with the moderately heavy workers falling in between. According to this study, the most active longshoremen doing the heaviest labour working in repeated bursts of peak activity, rather than at a steady, slow pace, were the most protected from heart attacks. In other words, the work habits of the heavy workers approximated the intensive exercise now thought to be a prevention of and protection against coronary heart disease.

How physical inactivity contributes to the development of coronary heart disease, and how intense physical activity protects against it, are not completely understood. There would be a simple explanation if it were true that physical inactivity, combined with high fat and cholesterol intake, promotes the development of atherosclerosis. In that case, intense daily physical activity that burned up fats and kept down body weight would prevent atherosclerosis. This theory could be accepted if heavy physical activity were at the same time to lower blood cholesterol concentration permanently. However, no significant lowering of the blood cholesterol concentration can be shown to result from heavy physical activity and exercise alone. And, since blood cholesterol has been shown to have a significant relationship to the development of atherosclerosis and heart attacks, it is difficult to explain this discrepancy.

There is no doubt, however, that physical activity has other beneficial effects in terms of heart and circulatory health. By dilating the small blood vessels in the muscles and the skin which are responsible for the resistance to blood flow, and thus the level of blood pressure, exercise will result in lowering of the blood pressure. Repeated constant heavy physical activity also improves the efficiency of the circulation by improving utilization of oxygen, by slowing the heart rate, and by increasing the force of the pumping chambers. It may also increase the calibre of the large coronary arteries, so that an obstructing plaque will have to grow much larger before it will significantly obstruct blood flow. Also, the communicating channels (called collateral arteries) between neighbouring blood vessels in the heart open up with heavy physical activity and, even if an obstruction develops, the damage is minimized by these collateral vessels shunting blood from the other major arteries towards the deprived area.

Exercise will also beneficially affect clotting mechanisms, and prevent the increased clotting tendencies often present in physically inactive people, which might also be a protecting factor in the physically active in the presence of an atherosclerotic plaque. And, finally, exercise and heavy physical activity have beneficial effects on the emotional balance of humans, generally promoting a feeling of overall well-being and an ability to cope with emotional stress with greater ease.

However, the state of medical knowledge at the present time is such that while we can make a case for heavy physical activity and regular heavy exercise as protecting against coronary heart disease, the mechanism by which physical inactivity may promote coronary heart disease and heart attacks is not known. Probably the most that can be fairly said is that physical inactivity is a permissive factor in the presence of other risk factors. On the other hand, there is no doubt that physical fitness and physical activity are important, in that, as we have seen, properly conducted physical activity has an important role in the comprehensive *overall* approach to the prevention of coronary heart disease.

To sum up, the causes of heart disease are multiple. As we have seen, a person can be born with a defective heart as a result of a metabolic disorder, or an infection of the mother during pregnancy. During life, and especially in early youth, a certain type of streptococcus infection (strep throat) can result in rheumatic fever that can damage the heart valves, causing them to function defectively. Later in life, virus infections, some metabolic disorders, and alcoholism can result in chronic heart muscle weakness. High blood pressure can tax the heart's ability to cope with the increased workload, eventually to the point of failure. And then, finally, there is coronary atherosclerosis – the major culprit. Coronary heart disease is by far the leading heart problem.

All of these problems will lead to one basic deficiency in

the heart's performance of its main life-giving function: pumping the blood to maintain an adequate circulation to all organs, in every circumstance of daily life.

We have indicated that, in all these cases, prevention is a better course of action than treatment of an already existing defect. The concept of prevention can be expanded to every cause of heart disease, including congenital heart disease, rheumatic heart disease, hypertension, and coronary heart disease. Medical science today possesses some truly miraculous treatments for some of these conditions, but this is a two-edged sword in that these processes through media exposure are often much more appealing to the public than the more simple measures of prevention.

Yet the hard fact is that, to eradicate heart disease, or at least markedly decrease its prevalence, much greater public awareness, education, and effort will be necessary than exist at the present time. Understanding of the causes and the risk factors, and willingness to make the effort to follow steps of prevention involving changes in life-style and attitude, are the keys to the problem.

3

The Symptoms of Heart Disease – True and False

It is amazing how misconceptions and old wives' tales persist in connection with human health. Today, despite great advances in medical techniques, wide availability of information, and excellent health care facilities, there are still plenty of misconceptions. Some of them are due to wilful ignorance or wishful thinking in order to avoid facing facts. Others are the result of self-interpretation, often biased by some controversial aspect of medicine widely publicized in the news media.

Even doctors can be bewildered by the disagreements among medical investigators, which sometimes cause them to avoid standing firm with patients and to let things ride until more definite information is available. It must be said that this attitude is sometimes justified in the interests of avoiding unnecessary worry, extremism, or excesses.

Individuals also often rationalize by accepting a misconception as a fact in order to avoid positive action. For instance, reports that some peasants in Soviet Georgia are enjoying fine health at ages in excess of 100 years while having been smokers all their lives, and similar misinterpreted scientific reports which show no relationship between cigarette smoking and lung cancer, are interpreted as proof of the harmlessness of smoking, despite the overwhelming evidence to the contrary.

As I indicated earlier, many myths and much of the mystery about heart disease have been eliminated during the last two centuries. However, some misconceptions still exist. For example, it is often believed that heredity plays such an overwhelming role in heart disease that no action can ever change a person's 'predetermination' to develop heart disease if his or her parents or grandparents have been so afflicted. As we explained in the previous chapter, heredity is only one of many interrelated factors which determine whether or not a person will develop heart disease. Many of these, when properly controlled, can suppress the role of heredity.

The myth that only high-level executives or people under the stress of intense business competition get heart attacks is rapidly fading, since so many people at all levels of society develop heart disease. Heart attacks are *not* the exclusive privilege of company presidents and top executives, but in fact hit at every level on the social scale almost equally from managers to blue collar workers.

It is often believed that tension and stress in daily life are the cause of heart attacks. Tension and stress have been with us since man has lived on earth, and they therefore cannot be singled out as the most important risk factor. It is true that a stressful and tension-filled life-style often is associated with particular habits that in themselves are leading risk factors. But, as we indicated earlier, classification of individuals by behavioural characteristics, and the relating of increased heart disease to a specific behavioural pattern (Type A), does not necessarily mean that the behavioural characteristic is the *primary* risk factor.

One of the most misunderstood problems – and one of the questions most frequently asked of doctors – is the meaning of the level of blood cholesterol as a risk factor. As we have seen earlier, the level of blood cholesterol has to be related to age, sex, and the presence or absence of other risk factors in order to be able to determine its risk score. In this context, it should be clearly stated that as low a level as possible should be everyone's goal, and especially the goal of those who possess other risk factors. This is possible by adopting particular eating habits, but it simply is not true that *all* fats and cholesterol have to be eliminated from the food in order to achieve that goal. A reasonable rearrangement of animal fats versus vegetable oils to control cholesterol intake will achieve the goal of a 'heart-saving' eating habit, and we shall show exactly how you can achieve that later in this book. At this point, all I would add is that there is no drug which can be easily taken to insure the achievement of this goal without following particular eating habits.

WARNING SIGNALS

There are early warning signals of heart disease, and there are also false signals. As so often in human behaviour, frequently we ignore the true warning signals while being over-concerned about the false signals. Let me therefore stress here that there is no way that you alone can determine the true meaning of a symptom or signal. To do so, you need the interpretation of an expert, your doctor.

In this context, let's consider for a moment the relatively frequent symptom of indigestion. Indigestion is usually the result of over-indulgence in eating, or of eating some improperly prepared or preserved food. All of us have on occasion experienced the heaviness in the stomach, heartburn, and nausea that follow food over-indulgence or the eating of spoiled food. Usually we recover after a day of fasting and rest, and the careful selection of light meals after the acute symptoms have subsided. Yet a feeling of indigestion can actually be an early sign of an impending heart attack. How can you be reasonably sure which of the two – upset stomach or impending heart attack – your symptoms of indigestion mean?

To answer that question, it is first essential to consider your age and sex. If you are a male under 30, or a female under 40, it is likely that symptoms of indigestion do really indicate an upset stomach and *not* a troubled heart. However, if the feeling of indigestion is different from any you have ever had before, or it changes its character during the first 30 minutes or hour, from a predominant pain in your stomach and nausea to pressure or heaviness in your chest radiating to your neck, then, whatever your age, you should not delay contacting your doctor. Do not be concerned about bothering him, because he would much rather you contact him as soon as such symptoms appear, particularly if you are a middle-aged or older male, or female past menopause. If you have no doctor, go to the emergency department of the hospital nearest to you.

Chest pain is one of the most characteristic and valuable symptoms in diagnosing coronary heart disease, but it is at the same time the most misunderstood symptom. There are some 101 different causes of chest pain, and coronary heart disease is only one of them. Actually, the description of this sensation as 'pain' is not always quite accurate, in that it is more often a heaviness, or sense of pressure, or a burning sensation behind the breast bone, left shoulder, or lower neck.

Often people are alarmed about short-lasting stabbing pains in the heart area which are severe enough to inhibit them from taking a deep breath. Such discomfort usually lasts only a few seconds, and at most less than a minute, and is unrelated to physical exertion or emotional excitement but often hits while sitting. Usually it improves with a few deep breaths, particularly forced exhaling. Most frequently this type of pain is the result of air located in the stomach or colon being trapped under the left diaphragm. Nervous eating and the consequent swallowing of excess air are often the cause. The feeling can be associated with jumping of the heart, or skipping beats and a feeling of palpitation.

Check with your doctor if such pains trouble you. A good physical examination usually will not only clear you as a suspect of heart disease, but allow your doctor to prescribe corrective measures – and to reassure you mentally.

Another form of chest pain that often causes people to

believe they have heart trouble is the type of pain connected with some form of physical stress or unusual physical activity recently performed. This can occur typically in a young mother who holds and carries around a baby of six months or more while trying to work with her other hand. Carrying such a weight in one arm, sweet as it may be, can put quite a strain on the arm, chest cage, and spine; and young mothers are frequent visitors to doctors' surgeries with complaints of pain in the centre of the chest. Typically, the pain is nagging, almost constant, and increases with movement of the arms; and, in the nervous tension created by caring for several young children simultaneously, mothers so afflicted often come to the doctor with real fears about heart disease. The pain is actually most often the result of a form of traumatic arthritis of one or more joints between the ribs and their vertebral bodies, and between the rib and the breast bone. It is increased by arm movements, and by slight pressure over the affected joints and their cartilage connections

Every individual doing unusual physical activities with his or her arms, or involving his or her chest cage, can have similar symptoms of pain in the chest wall, and it is often interpreted as pain from the heart. The appropriate action is to let your doctor determine the nature of the pain, reassure you if, as most likely, it is simply muscular in origin, and in addition prescribe some effective remedies.

Another form of chest pain, arising from what is commonly known as 'pinched nerve', results in tensing of the muscles between the ribs, and is a form of nerve irritation called intercostal neuralgia. This type of pain usually is quite severe, increases with movement of the chest or deep breathing, and persists for several days. It responds to rest and medications that reduce inflammation of the nerve and muscle.

Despite its many different forms and causes, as we have said, the symptom of chest pain is one of the most valuable diagnostic signs available to the doctor in suspecting and diagnosing coronary heart disease. True angina has several typical characteristics which differentiate it from other causes of chest pain. Usually the discomfort is, as we have said, more a feeling of pressure or 'heaviness' behind the breast bone, or a burning or ache between the shoulder blades, sometimes radiating to the neck, the jaw, the left shoulder, and the inner area of the upper arm down to the elbow. Initially, it occurs during or following exertion or excitement, lasts 30 seconds to a few minutes, and subsides during rest or calming down. It often occurs in the morning when walking quickly in cold weather, and sometimes during the night when awakening from sleep. The initial discomfort can sometimes subside when the physical activity is continued, and this is called the 'walk-through pain'. This type of discomfort can be fairly minimal and increase neither in severity nor frequency, or it can get progressively worse.

Such type of chest discomfort definitely requires a good physical examination for full evaluation. There are excellent methods of diagnosing the cause of the condition, such as properly prescribed treadmill exercise tests, or continuous recording of the electrocardiogram on a tape recorder during various activities of the day for subsequent analysis.

Even before the occurrence of such definite symptoms as chest pain or shortness of breath, there are other signals or warnings of heart disease in many individuals. But in many instances these warnings may not be manifested in specific symptoms and thus can go unnoticed until they are eventually detected by medical examination. That is why it pays to have regular check-ups.

We have discussed in detail how coronary heart disease and heart attacks are enhanced by so-called specific risk factors. Doctors today can actually estimate the risk of developing heart disease or heart attack in any individual in, let us say, the next six years, by determining his or her risk score or profile.

If you are in business and you are planning an investment, you evaluate, if you are wise, the risk factors of that investment. You analyse the different aspects of the proposition, the overall economic climate, your chances of return, your risk of losing your investment, and so on. In other words, you construct a 'return and risk profile' of your investment. And you would consider extremely foolish anyone who would make an investment without such an evaluation, or who would invest against a large risk factor with little or no chance of a fair return. Why is it, then, that many people do not apply the same principles when investing in their own health and life?

Many individuals – including even the cleverest business people – do not obtain such an evaluation of their health and their heart attack 'risk profile'. And even when they do have a thorough medical examination and an evaluation of their health and warning signals are indicated to them, many often do not even then follow whatever instructions are given them to correct the problem. In other words, they make, at best, an unwise, and, at worst, a downright foolish investment with their health.

There are several warning signals which can double, triple, or multiply by a factor of 10 or even 20 the risk of developing heart disease or heart attack in the years ahead, just as there are warning signals that can indicate a business venture beginning to turn catastrophic.

Overweight is one of the most frequent and simplest of these warning signals. We have seen that overweight is often associated with increased blood pressure and elevated blood cholesterol, both of which are very strong risk factors. If, then, in addition, there is a family history of diabetes or a tendency towards heart disease, and all this is topped by heavy smoking, the unfavourable conditions are so greatly increased that the risk may well become 10 to 20 times greater than average. Since the average is calculated as the average British risk (normal blood pressure, no cigarette smoking, and average British cholesterol level), the average risk to the British is already high compared with that to the

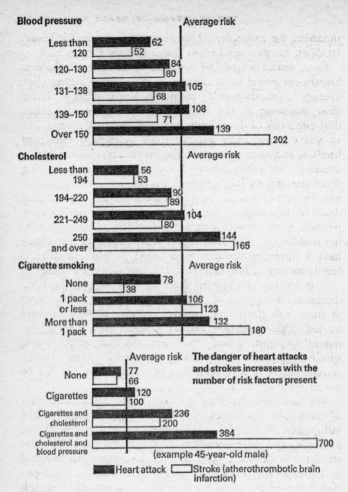

Blood pressure

Less than 120: 62 / 52
120–130: 84 / 80
131–138: 105 / 68
139–150: 108 / 71
Over 150: 139 / 202

Cholesterol

Less than 194: 56 / 53
194–220: 90 / 89
221–249: 104 / 80
250 and over: 144 / 165

Cigarette smoking

None: 78 / 38
1 pack or less: 106 / 123
More than 1 pack: 132 / 180

None: 77 / 66
Cigarettes: 120 / 100
Cigarettes and cholesterol: 236 / 200
Cigarettes and cholesterol and blood pressure: 384 / 700

Average risk

The danger of heart attacks and strokes increases with the number of risk factors present

(example 45-year-old male)

■ Heart attack □ Stroke (atherothrombotic brain infarction)

The effect of high blood pressure, blood cholesterol and cigarette smoking on risk of heart attack and stroke. The higher the blood pressure (from left to right), cholesterol and number of cigarettes smoked per day, the higher is the risk. Presence of all three (lower graph) in an individual multiplies the risk several times.

Source: The Framingham, Mass., Heart Study

Japanese, for example, whose average cholesterol is lower. In short, the average British risk is already far too high.

Now, would anyone of a sound mind make a business investment based on a risk 20 or more times higher than average? Nobody would, of course. Yet the fact is that a clear warning, as the result of a medical examination, that one's risk of developing heart disease in the next 6 or 12 years is markedly greater than average is often not heeded; and even when it is, the instructions for corrective measures are often followed half-heartedly at best. Yet, these warning signals, although maybe not yet incapacitating, are just as real as the warning signals of a bad business deal. In this respect, it is simply common sense to have periodic medical check-ups, particularly if you are approaching middle-age, if you know you are overweight, if you may have a tendency towards high blood pressure, if there is family history of heart disease, and if you are a smoker.

It is not my purpose to describe fully here the various diagnostic symptoms of cardiovascular disease, since most of them will move you by their nature to seek medical advice. The important factors are the *early signs of increased risk*, even though they may not yet be producing specific symptoms. However, a few words about specific warning signs of an impending heart attack might not be out of place at this point.

We have already outlined the different characteristics of chest pain. Sometimes a mild episode of discomfort like indigestion or heartburn is followed by extreme tiredness, lassitude, and depression for several days before a second similar episode leads to a heart attack. Thus any unusual and unexplained occurrence of chest discomfort and indigestion, followed by weakness, paleness, and lassitude – especially in a middle-aged male or post-menopausal female – should have immediate medical attention, because thereby a major heart attack may be prevented, or its impact minimized. In these circumstances, do not hesitate to ring your doctor and fully describe your symptoms to him, so that he can immediately initiate diagnostic tests. Such a call may save your life.

I realize that the much-publicized problem of heart disease may create unnecessary worries and even hypochondria in some individuals. However, so-called 'psychosomatic' heart disease – the experiencing of symptoms of heart disease by imagining them – is usually triggered by misunderstanding of a doctor's remarks, or misinterpretation of his or her actions, rather than by the general national campaign to prevent heart disease. If you have any misgivings or fears about the condition of your heart or your health generally, you should, without hesitation, ask your doctor to explain your condition to you. Usually he or she will tell you exactly what you should know about your problem. If you feel that you have not received a full explanation, don't hesitate to indicate this to your physician, and to continue to request it until you have a full understanding of your condition.

ASSOCIATED DISEASES

I explained earlier how the heart and circulatory system are closely tied together functionally. This is true not only of the physiological function of the system, but also in terms of disease, in that malfunction of any individual part of the system will affect the function of the whole. In other words, the two major heart disease problems – atherosclerosis and high blood pressure – can manifest themselves in other organ disease, such as kidney disease, obstruction of blood flow to the legs, stroke, etc.

When an obstructing plaque is located in an artery supplying blood to the brain, the obstruction of blood flow can result in clotting of blood in that artery. This is the most frequent cause of a stroke. More rarely, a stroke can be caused by a rupture of an artery of the brain when the external wall is weakened by marked hypertension. A ruptured artery is more often fatal, as blood clots frequently can be dissolved and partial or complete function of the damaged nerve centres restored.

In some instances, blood flow to the brain is temporarily decreased in the presence of an obstructing plaque, resulting in brief episodes of impaired function of certain brain centres. This causes temporary disorientation (or 'passing out'), weakness or paralysis of an arm and leg on one side of the body, speech difficulty, and so on. If the obstructing plaque can be localized by diagnostic studies, it may be surgically removed and circulation to the brain restored. This condition is called cerebral vascular insufficiency; or carotid artery insufficiency, when the carotid artery, one of the main arteries supplying the brain, is obstructed.

When the arteries to one or both of the legs are obstructed by a plaque, the blood flow to the leg muscles is insufficient and severe pain in the calf or the entire leg will develop during walking. Typically, the pain disappears after a few minutes of rest. If the obstruction is more severe, and located more upstream in the arterial system, visible paleness and coldness of the skin, together with pain, can be present even at rest. By localizing the plaque by diagnostic tests, the circulation to the leg often can be restored by surgical bypass of the obstruction using a dacron graft.

When an obstructing plaque develops in the artery supplying blood to one of the kidneys, a curious mechanism is stimulated in that kidney: the physiological mechanism regulating water and salt metabolism to maintain normal blood pressure is falsely activated. Since the obstruction to blood flow will decrease blood pressure beyond the obstruction, pressure-sensitive nerve endings in the small blood vessels of the kidney, acting in response to the false signal that the blood pressure is too low, will stimulate the release of an enzyme called renin. Renin will then combine with a factor of the blood from the liver and together they will produce the vasoconstrictor, angiotensin. This substance will stimulate excessive salt (sodium) and water retention and constriction of small arteries, which in turn will increase the blood pressure. If hypertension existed prior to the obstruction of the kidney artery, the blood pressure will further increase.

This renal form of hypertension is present in approximately 10 per cent of all cases of high blood pressure. When it is recognized and diagnosed, the high blood pressure can in many cases be cured or improved by removing the plaque, or by bypassing the obstruction through surgical means.

Sometimes high blood pressure significantly damages the small arteries of the kidney. This may result in kidney failure and a malignant form of hypertension with kidney disease called nephrosclerosis. In these cases, malfunction of the kidneys will lead to lack of elimination of metabolic by-products and poisoning of the blood. Only heroic measures, such as kidney dialysis and kidney transplant, will then prolong life.

All of the foregoing disease conditions, including heart attack, occur in the end stage of the long process of atherosclerosis. Unfortunately, atherosclerosis cannot be diagnosed in any of its forms *before* it produces symptoms, and this is the main reason why atherosclerosis is such a devastating disease. It sneaks up on you if you are not on your guard, which is why I cannot stress too strongly the importance of correcting risk factors to improve your risk score before symptoms of disease in any of your vulnerable organs do occur.

It is not yet known what factors in an individual determine where in the circulatory system an atherosclerotic plaque will develop. Thus it is impossible to predict whether the heart (coronary arteries), the brain, the kidneys, the legs, or other organs will be affected by the atherosclerotic process. Atherosclerosis is often present in more than one artery, and symptoms will occur first in the organ which is affected most by the blood-flow obstruction.

Sometimes people who have had problems with circulation to their legs may later suffer heart attacks or strokes. Thus, the consequences of atherosclerosis are mostly unpredictable.

4

Treatment and Research

The greatest advances in the treatment and prevention of
heart and vascular diseases have been made in the last 30
years. This is not to say, however, that great advances did
not take place prior to 1945. As a matter of fact, all the
recent advances were made possible by the dedicated pio-
neers of the preceding decades of this century and the two
or more previous centuries. But our understanding of
disease and methods of treatment accelerated almost
exponentially after the Second World War, as the result of
great research efforts aided by massive advances in technology and the generous support given by society and
governments to promote the cause of better health.

We have seen that prevention is always a better course
of action than treatment of an already existing heart or
other organic disease. Since heart attack, stroke, kidney
malfunction, etc., are the *end* stages of atherosclerosis and
hypertension, prevention of the development or progression
of atherosclerosis and hypertension is by far the most
effective form of 'treatment'. And, thanks to unceasing
research efforts, we have now very effective preventive
measures and treatments.

High blood pressure may cause absolutely no symptoms
in its early stage, and thus may easily escape early treatment unless detected by physical examination. Yet it has
been shown by the Veterans Administration Cooperative
Research Group in the United States that treatment of even
mild forms of hypertension will decrease the incidence of
strokes and heart attacks in subsequent years. Therefore,
the treatment of even the mildest high blood pressure,

which does not cause any symptoms (is asymptomatic), is fully justifiable as a preventive measure. Fortunately, many doctors agree with this concept and today treat mild asymptomatic hypertension as carefully as other ills. Their job is made easier than in the past by the existence of very effective drugs that have minimal side effects, due to the continuing efforts of researchers and the pharmaceutical industry.

When hypertension becomes so severe that the so-called 'first-line' drugs become ineffective, more effective drugs or drug combinations are available, many of which have been developed and tested only in the past ten years. Naturally, the higher the blood pressure and the more stubborn its response to treatment, the stronger the drug or drug combination needed for effective treatment, and the higher the incidence of side effects. However, we have such effective drugs today that anybody's blood pressure can be lowered to normal. The problem is not so much to achieve that level as to go slowly enough to avoid serious side effects from the rapid lowering itself, and from the side effects of drugs.

Some 20 years ago, attempts were made to lower blood pressure by surgically disrupting the nerve roots along the vertebral bodies in the chest which innervate the blood vessels and control the calibre of the small arteries. This technique, developed by Dr Smithwick at Harvard, lowered the blood pressure in a large percentage of the patients so treated. However, the patients had a tendency to faint when standing, and their blood pressure tended to creep up again some years later because the nerves had a great tendency to reconnect, control the blood vessels again, and thereby send up the blood pressure. With the advance of newly effective drugs, the Smithwick operation was discarded.

The emphasis in this book being on the *prevention* of heart and circulatory disease, it must be said that identification of the so-called risk factors, and definite proof that they separately and in combination enhance the disease process, is comparatively recent. Indeed, methods of preventive treatment are actually being tested on a large scale only at the present time. However, there are already a number of reports which show that effective reduction of the risk factors have resulted in regression of the atherosclerotic process and improvement of the symptoms. In fact, from these reports it appears that, even after recovery from a heart attack, risk factor reduction seems to be effective in preventing further attacks.

Research over the past ten years has shown that there are different inherited and acquired abnormalities in the metabolism of blood fats and cholesterol. Fat particles are transported in the blood bound chemically to protein molecules. Depending on the size of the molecules so formed – called lipoprotein – electrically charged lipoprotein molecules will, in a test tube, travel slower or faster in an electric field. By this so-called electrophoresis technique, different distribution of the different-size lipoprotein molecules can be achieved.

In some individuals, there is an abnormal distribution, which has been arbitrarily divided into five recognizable lipoprotein abnormalities. Some of these abnormalities are inherited, while others are acquired, and the tendency to atherosclerosis and heart attacks varies between very high to very low in these cases. In some conditions, in addition to dietary restriction of fat and cholesterol, drug treatment is necessary to correct the abnormality. However, in most individuals, restriction of animal fat and cholesterol intake is sufficient to lower blood cholesterol and to modify lipoprotein abnormality.

There are conflicting results when drugs alone are used without dietary restriction to lower cholesterol levels. Even when the drug has reduced the blood cholesterol level, in a recent study the recurrence of heart attacks was not lower in the drug-treated group than in an untreated control group. On the other hand, a previous study suggested that in a large group of individuals treated with an anti-cholesterol agent, the incidence of the first heart attack was lower than in the untreated group in a six-year observation period. Further studies are needed to test the blood-cholesterol-lowering effect of drugs alone, without dietary modification, and to correlate it with the reduction, if any, in heart attacks.

The present massive efforts to salvage and improve the function of the heart and vascular system after damage by heart attack or stroke will continue. Survival of heart attack victims, after appropriate medical help, has improved markedly over the past 15 years. The introduction of the coronary care unit system, new drugs that prevent cardiac arrest, and new techniques of resuscitation are among the factors that have markedly improved the survival rate of hospitalized heart attack patients in the first 24 to 48 hours.

More than half of the deaths from heart attacks, however, occur in the initial hours before medical help is obtained. One reason this toll remains so heavy is that early symptoms of heart attack are often not recognized by either the afflicted or those around them. Another reason is that, even when the symptoms are recognized, tremendous logistical problems must often be surmounted to move the patient fast enough to a properly equipped medical facility or to apply resuscitation measures. Pre-hospital care problems are being studied presently, and it is to be hoped that this research will improve the deficiencies of the system.

When an individual has survived the initial phase of a heart attack and is recovering in the coronary care unit, various supportive measures are available to the doctors to help nature to heal the damage with the least possible incapacitation of the patient. And, of course, there is a continuing massive research effort to find even better methods of treatment, in order to salvage as much heart muscle tissue as possible, and to retain as much cardiovascular function as possible after recovery from the attack.

Some promising new treatments to be applied in the

initial phase of a heart attack have just been introduced on a trial basis, but it is too early as yet to predict how effective they will be.

After recovery from a heart attack, preventive measures against further atherosclerosis become vitally important, and must be started immediately if they had not already been introduced before the attack. These measures include drugs, psychological support, and rehabilitation with programmed physical activity, and they have greatly improved the treatment and the outlook of many heart attack victims.

There are, unfortunately, still insufficient rehabilitation programmes and facilities for post-hospital care of the large number of British heart attack victims. But there is also much that can be done by the individual for himself, with the guidance of his doctor and a little self-discipline. Indeed, the one piece of good news for heart attack victims is that most people who survive and recover from an attack return to a happy and productive life.

LOOKING INTO THE FUTURE

We are enjoying today the fruits of the relentless research efforts of the past and of our own intensely research-oriented time. Advances in technology have given us tools of a once unthinkable nature that permit accuracy and reliability in probing the inside of the heart and the vascular system, open-heart surgery, atomic-powered pacemakers, artificial valves, artificial blood vessels, artificial hearts, and so on – the list is endless. Advances in the basic sciences have helped us to understand the biochemistry and metabolism of bacteria and viruses, and have led to the identification of antidotes and, through these, the eradication of almost all infectious diseases. The discovery of the ultrastructure and biochemistry of the cell nucleus and its major components, RNA and DNA, and their biosynthesis, have brought us closer to full understanding of cell metabolism, which brings us gradually closer to the solution of the cancer mystery.

In the area of heart disease, our knowledge about the biochemistry of the heart muscle and its contraction has increased enormously, as has knowledge that brings closer the solution to atherosclerosis. For example, high blood pressure is better understood, and the identification of its cause cannot be too far away with the present pace of research.

But even when we will be able to organize rescue systems that salvage more heart attack victims before they reach hospitals, or find better means of treatment in the first few hours of heart attacks, or learn how to salvage even more heart muscle for future function, or develop better artificial blood vessels, heart valves, bypass grafts, pacemakers, artificial hearts, and so on, I have to emphasize and re-emphasize that heart attacks, strokes, vascular obstructions, kidney disease, etc., are *end stages* of the long process of atherosclerosis and hypertension. Because that is and always will be so, people will never be saved from these afflictions by pills, or operations, or pacemakers, or even by artificial hearts. In the end, all that will save them is their own self-love and self-respect, as these determine their individual day to day life styles. In short, *the future is in prevention.*

While we must sustain maximum effort to salvage already damaged hearts, our greatest future effort should be in prevention: in making the means of prevention known and available to everyone, and in increasing the effectiveness of methods of prevention. Prevention can be practised, once he or she knows how, by every human being. *You can do it yourself*, whereas you cannot treat yourself and cure yourself after you have become ill.

It is my conviction that there cannot be too much effort in the techniques of prevention. These efforts must transcend the purely medical factors. They must one day, for example, make 'preventing eating' easy for individuals by means of food and restaurant industry policies that make selection of heart-saving foods readily accessible, even though this may mean restraining the taste buds of Britons and other peoples whose eating habits are killing them. In like manner, the harmfulness of tobacco must be studied to the point where the mechanism of its damaging effects is so completely exposed that elimination of the habit becomes demanded by everyone.

Because the effect of stress on heart and vascular disease is not well understood, it too requires intensive and continuing investigation to uncover the exact relationships of psychological makeup, behaviour characteristics, and outside stress factors on heart disease. In this region there is a rather interesting field which has had very little attention in the past, called biofeedback, which indicates that conditioned reflexes may operate as part of a vicious cycle in heart and other disease mechanisms.

The mechanism of ageing will also be studied more extensively in the future, because it is not sufficient simply to prolong life, but also necessary to improve physical and mental capacities for fuller enjoyment of life in older age. A better understanding of the ageing process, its prevention and treatment, will achieve that goal, along with the psycho-social relationships of ageing that will also be explored in greater detail in the future.

All of this will, then, become part of a great preventive effort which, in the final analysis, will have to achieve the goal of improved health for all people by public education. And I believe it will happen, because only a combined and massive effort in all these fields will have the greatest benefit to our national health with reasonable cost effectiveness.

PART TWO

The Factors that Affect Your Heart

5

Your Sex and Your Heart

Men and women on the whole do not differ significantly in either the function of their hearts or their susceptibility to heart disease. There are, however, some minor differences between them in these regards:

Women, on the average, have somewhat smaller hearts than men. The normal resting heart rate is on the average slightly higher in women than in men, and the amount of blood ejected with each beat (stroke volume) is slightly smaller. The maximum heart rate which can be reached during heavy exercise, the maximum amount of blood returned in the circulation in a minute (cardiac output), and the maximum oxygen uptake (the amount of oxygen consumed in a minute during heavy exercise) are on the average slightly higher in men than in women. Otherwise, all functions are very similar. Women can be trained as athletes just as well as men, but, because of body constitution, their peak performance will be on the average somewhat below that of men – although this is not to say that certain women athletes' peak cardiac performances will not exceed that of many male athletes. What differences there are in heart performance between men and women are attributable to differences in the ratio of muscle mass to body weight, and, on the whole, to smaller body frame and height.

There are also minor differences between men and women in regard to heart disease. Some of these differences relate to genetic factors, others to environmental influences, and still others to differences in the influence of sex hormones on the development of heart disease. There are certain congenital heart conditions that are transmitted in sex chromosomes (genes transmitting sex characteristics), but these are relatively rare. Rheumatic heart disease seems to be slightly more prevalent in women than in men, and women suffering from this condition more often have involvement of the mitral valve (the valve between the left atrium and the left ventricle), while in men the aortic valve (the valve between the aorta and the left pumping chamber) is more often involved. The cause of this difference is not known, but, since the difference is minor, it has, from the medical standpoint, very little practical significance.

High blood pressure, arteriosclerosis, and coronary heart disease have some sex-related differences in their evolutionary course. Some women have a tendency to accumulate fluids just prior to menstruation and a tendency to slightly increased blood pressure during this time. Also, some women respond to oral contraceptives with water retention and blood-pressure increase – both changes being related to the sex hormones and their effect on the body's handling of fluids and salt (sodium).

The increased tendency of women to develop high blood pressure after the menopause appears to be related more to their tendency to increasing body weight than to the change in sex hormones arising from the menopause. As we have seen, there is a definite relationship between overweight and the tendency to high blood pressure, and weight reduction alone is often a very effective means of reducing hypertension. The cause of the increased tendency to obesity in women after the menopause is complex and can be explained only partially by changes in sex hormone production. Psychological effects of menopause may result in overeating and decreased physical activity, which are probably just as important as hormonal changes, if not more so. The age-related decrease in distensibility of the vascular system is probably aggravated by overweight. This, in concert with the hormonally created water and salt imbalance, can result in a tendency to elevation of the blood pressure and eventually to hypertension. In men the same processes work, but more slowly. Hypertension is often increasingly present in overweight men as they get older.

Certain forms of hypertension may show some variations in males and females, but the significance of these differences in the context of this discussion is minimal. It has been observed, for example, that a specific muscular growth can obstruct the renal arteries and lead to marked elevation of the blood pressure, and this is more common in young females than in males (in both cases the condition can be cured by surgery). So-called malignant hypertension, a severe form of high blood pressure, seems to progress more rapidly in males than in females. However, all these conditions are relative rarities and are mentioned here only for completeness.

Beyond these factors there is, however, a definite sex-related difference in the development of general arteriosclerosis and atherosclerotic coronary heart disease. Until recently, coronary heart disease and myocardial infarction were relatively rare in women before the menopause, whereas in males the incidence showed a gradual increase with age. This observation led investigators to study the effect of sex hormones on the development of atherosclerosis. The famous studies of the late Louis Katz and his co-workers at the Michael Reese Research Institute of Chicago, some 20 years ago, showed that the development of arteriosclerosis produced in chicks, caused by feeding them a high cholesterol and fat diet, could be prevented by administration of the female sex hormone oestrogen. This led to the speculation that females are protected from the development of atherosclerosis before menopause by their own oestrogen produced in the ovaries, which was thought possibly to account for the relative rarity of coronary heart disease in females before the menopause. This possibility is supported by the fact that no such protection seems to be present in women in whom the ovaries were removed prior to menopause; indeed, in ovarectomized

women the frequency of coronary heart disease appears to
be similar to that of men in the different age groups.

Basing their work on the studies of Dr Katz and his colleagues, doctors attempted to treat already existing severe
atherosclerosis in males with the female sex hormone oestrogen. However, no definite beneficial effect could be observed, and the side effects of feminization – enlargement
and tenderness of the breasts, decreased sexual function,
impotence, etc. – prevented the widespread application of
the treatment. Thus it was rapidly replaced by the discovery of other means of decreasing risk factors, and the
availability of other treatments.

Women are often treated with oestrogen in the menopause, and thereafter, to decrease the impact of change
in sexual hormone activity and to soften the transition
from the menstrual stage to the postmenstrual stage, a
practice which probably to some degree extends the protective effect of sex hormones against atherosclerosis in
women. The protection of female hormones, however,
would seem in itself to be limited, since recently an increase of coronary heart disease and heart attacks has been
reported in young women in the premenopausal phase of
life. Probably two factors are mainly responsible for this:
first, the increased cigarette smoking in women and its
earlier commencement, and, second, the increased social
and work pressures on women as they enter more competi-
tively into the job market. Clearly, whatever the specific
causes, any protective effect of female sex hormones is overcome by increased exposure to strong risk factors, a price
which many women now seem to be willing to pay for their
much-coveted liberation. In the future, as a consequence,
we will undoubtedly see less of a difference in the incidence
of coronary heart disease between males and premenopausal females.

6

Your Heredity and Your Heart

We have already alluded to the fact that heredity has a role in the risk of heart disease. The question is, of course, how *strong* a role does heredity play?

The influence of heredity has been studied in the different heart conditions by examining family members through the construction of family heredity trees, by identical and non-identical twin studies, by comparing ethnic and racial groups, and by many other means. Rather than go fully into the results of these studies, our purpose in this book would be best served by an overview of heredity as it is viewed today in some of the most important heart problems, and by elimination of some of the misconceptions about it which exist in the minds of many people.

Heredity plays an important role in determining our constitution, our body build, our appearance, and, within limits, the functioning of our cardiovascular system. Heredity is charted by the genes contained in the chromosomes present in every nucleus of our body cells.

The genes in the chromosomes of the egg (ovum) from your mother and the seed (sperm cell) from your father contained the characteristics that caused you to be what you are. A combination of these characteristics from the line of your mother and father, after fertilization of the ovum by the sperm, resulted in a combination of characteristics which is special to you and you alone. This is why children can have combinations of characteristics which do not completely duplicate their father or mother, or any of their ancestors. Body build, body function, psychological makeup, mental ability, etc., are an unpredictable mixture of the characteristics of your entire ancestry. Topping this, of course, is the strong modifying effect of your environment, which cannot be neglected when analysing either your physical or psychological makeup. Many children when they grow up behave like one or both of their parents not only because of their inherited characteristics, but also because of habits resulting from environmental influences imparted by their parents.

What does this have to do with your heart? The answer is – a lot.

Whether or not you become an athlete, a businessman, a scientist, an artist, a salesman, a blue-collar worker, or whatever – and whether or not you will be a physically or mentally active or lazy individual, an over-indulger or a moderate and sensible eater or drinker, a creative or an intellectually dull individual, an emotionally balanced or imbalanced person, and so on – depends on multiple interrelated factors where inheritance, environmental family ties, and luck play a greater or smaller role in a whole series of combinations. In the same way, whether or not one of us has developed a strong athletic cardiovascular system cannot be laid entirely at the door of heredity. Environment has a very significant role in what we make of and do to ourselves, by motivating and stimulating us to develop ourselves even in the face of less than average inherited physical constitution or mental capacity. Similarly, the resistance to heart disease is greatly influenced by outside factors. For example, a fatalistic and gloomy outlook, born of the belief that heredity must inevitably cause a person to be miserable, is often only an excuse for relinquishing personal responsibility in governing our fate.

Let us then in this light see if we can identify the truth about heredity and heart disease.

We discussed earlier a group of heart conditions known as congenital heart disease: diseases that are either hereditary by genetic transmission, or are due to intrauterine (prior to birth) damage, usually an arrest in the development of the heart and circulatory system. We have seen that the chance of congenital heart disease may be decreased by genetic counselling or preventive measures during intrauterine development. Overall, we have seen that the number of *congenital* heart conditions is relatively small.

The role of heredity in the far more prevalent high blood pressure and coronary heart disease is a much more mysterious question, and especially its effect on those who have apparently been bestowed with a normal heart and vascular system at birth. In fact, it is mysterious enough for us to have to ask ourselves whether heredity really has as strong a role as believed by many in the development of these diseases.

When doctors take a medical history at the time of your physical examination, they routinely ask you about your father and mother, and your other ancestors – basically, whether or not they have or had high blood pressure or heart disease. It is not difficult in these circumstances for a certain type of person to make an internal, fatalistic conclusion that sure enough his father or mother had high blood pressure, or his uncle died of a heart attack, or whatever, and that he therefore is predestined by fate to the same affliction. Such a gloomy conclusion is not justified, and is never the intent of the inquiry by a doctor. As we stressed earlier, hereditary factors are perhaps only some of many, many among the complex aetiology of hypertensive and coronary heart disease. Even the so-called familial hyperlipidemia (a form of abnormal cholesterol and fat metabolism frequent in members of certain families), with its high incidence of coronary heart disease, is only *one* of the risk factors. Proper diet can quite effectively correct this cholesterol abnormality and thereby greatly reduce the risk of coronary heart disease.

Studies of hereditary factors in identical and non-identical twins have shown that inheritance appears to have only a moderate determining influence on whether or not an individual will develop high blood pressure or coronary heart disease. In fact, *all* other arteriosclerotic vascular diseases, such as strokes, etc., are caused by *multiple* interrelated factors acting collectively. That is the reason why one cannot simply blame *one* factor, such as overeating, or physical inactivity, or heredity, or smoking, or frustration, or Type A behaviour, for heart disease. Prevention lies in reducing *all* the most unfavourable factors we can do something about, of which there is a long list. The fortunate thing is that we can rank these factors in order of importance and attack the most hazardous ones most vigorously in order to achieve effective and lasting prevention. And heredity, which admittedly we cannot attack, occupies a position of only medium importance in this long list of risk factors.

Don't therefore be despondent about heredity, and don't use it as a crutch to excuse yourself from making a rewarding effort to modify the modifiable risk factors. Recognize that it is rarely heredity alone that causes heart disease, but the *combined influence* of many other factors about which you can take definite preventive action.

7

Your Age and Your Heart

Peak performance in athletes is usually reached in the early twenties and maintained until the late twenties. But this can vary with different sports. For example, women may win their first Olympic medals in swimming, gymnastics, and ice skating in their teens, whereas men usually seem to win theirs in their early twenties. Peak performance in these sports may decline in the mid and late twenties, respectively. In other types of sports, peak performance sometimes lasts into the forties.

The limiting factor in sports performance is predominantly the function of the cardiovascular system. With adequate training, it can maintain its peak performance for many years, but there inevitably occurs an age-related cardiovascular decline both in athletes and non-athletes. How does this age-related decline affect different individuals?

I have seen men and women in their mid seventies and early eighties perform acrobatic, gymnastic, and athletic activities that would be to the credit of a 20-year-old. What is their secret? In addition to a strong inherited constitution, *it is beyond question the result of systematic and continued exercise and a prudent life based on moderation and the avoidance of all excesses.*

While the possibility of a healthful, active, and useful old age exists for all of us, as we have said, the cardiovascular system does show some changes with advancing age. Along with all of our body tissues, the walls of the blood vessels start to lose their elasticity, just like an ageing rubber hose. Exactly when these changes begin differs widely among individuals. The study of ageing is a science in it-self, and scientists have gained some insight in recent years into some of the factors determining the rate of ageing. However, we are far away as yet from knowing all the mechanisms of ageing, and thus from starting effective and systematic prevention and treatment programmes against early ageing. The eternal-youth serum has not yet been dis-covered.

It is a known fact that blood pressure increases with age. We used to say that 100 plus your age for your systolic blood pressure is a 'normal' increase. Thus, a 60-year-old person may have a 'normal' systolic blood pressure of 160 mm Hg, with the diastolic pressure changed very little or perhaps slightly increased. This was thought to be due to the loss of elasticity of the largest blood vessel, the aorta, in that the energy produced by the heart during systolic contraction will raise the blood pressure higher in the presence of a stiff aorta than in a more elastic vessel. However, we soon learned that what we considered a normal age-adjusted increase of the blood pressure in the Western world may not be true for natives of India, China, and parts of Africa. In other words, different populations show vast differences in the rate at which elasticity of the vascular system is lost with ageing. And, clearly, among nations with very little or no increase of the systolic blood pressure with age, the vas-cular system maintains its youthful elasticity for a much longer period than in a population with increasing blood pressure such as ours. While not all the answers are now available to explain these differences, one of the factors behind the earlier loss of arterial elasticity in the Western civilization is earlier arteriosclerosis.

Today the belief that your blood pressure is normal when you add your age to the number 100 is no longer valid. In fact, most physicians today consider abnormal an elevation of the systolic blood pressure above 140 mm Hg, and of the diastolic blood pressure above 90 mm Hg in the resting state. (It should be noted, however, that measurement of a higher blood pressure on one occasion only should not be considered as an indication of high blood pressure.)

What all this basically means is that the ageing of your cardiovascular system can be vastly different from that of your contemporaries, depending on many factors. In short, you can maintain the youthfulness of your cardiovascular system by proper living – which we will discuss later – even without the availability of a rejuvenating serum.

It might be appropriate here to mention again the difference in men and women in the age-related development of atherosclerosis and coronary heart disease. We have already indicated that women seem to be protected to a certain degree from early atherosclerosis and coronary heart disease during the age range of their normal menstrual cycle. After the menopause, when the protective effect of the oestrogens has ceased, women catch up with men very quickly, and in the sixth decade these differences in the susceptibility to coronary heart disease disappear. However, if present trends continue and women continue to expose themselves earlier to risk factors other than age, the differences in incidence in heart attacks between men and women in the younger age groups will be narrowed in the future. Also, in men we now see the development of coronary heart disease at ever earlier ages. It was at one time the disease of the middle and older age groups, but heart attacks in men in their twenties are nowadays not unfamiliar to practising doctors.

The clear message here is that, while age and ageing have a considerable effect on the performance of your heart and vascular system – and thus on the risk of heart disease – it is not so much age *per se* as *early ageing* that is the greatest hazard. And this you can delay to a considerable degree, if you are determined to do so.

8

Your Physique and Your Heart

Your constitution, or 'physique', is determined by heredity and then modified, as we have seen earlier, by your life style, and the interrelationship is complex.

The characteristics of your constitution are your height, body configuration, weight, muscle mass, facial appearance, metabolism (within certain limits), emotional characteristics, cardiovascular function and responses, and ultimately your susceptibility to heart and vascular diseases.

It is generally considered that height is a constitutional characteristic, and that differences in height and body build are transmitted by racial heredity: in other words, both the tall, Nordic peoples and the relatively smaller people of the Far East, parts of Africa, and most Mediterranean countries inherit their build from their ancestors. Yet it is not quite that simple.

Height is the result of bone growth stimulated by the growth hormone of the pituitary gland, and depends upon how much growth occurs before the bone growth factory cells (present in the end portions of each bone) terminate their function. The amount of protein in the food is one factor that determines the production of growth hormone and bone growth, and it has been shown that low protein intake in childhood can result in relatively low adult height. This would seem to be borne out by the fact that increased adoption of Western-style eating habits and economic growth since the Second World War have led to a considerable increase in the average height of young people in Japan, a nation well known for its low average height. Thus, height as a constitutional characteristic transmitted by heredity can at times be modified by external factors.

The same is true of other constitutional characteristics. Psychological makeup and emotional response to stress are partly constitutional, but to a large extent they are also the result of cultural background, national and social trends, and family and other ties. For example, Rosenman and Friedman, in a study of the psychological makeup of Japanese-Americans, found that Japanese living in the United States who remained true to their cultural customs and family ties were similar to Japanese living in Japan in terms of the preponderance of Type As and Type Bs, with Type As being quite rare. Correspondingly, these Japanese have a lower incidence of coronary heart disease than the American average. On the other hand, Japanese who have adopted Western-style living and customs approached distribution between Type As and Type Bs similar to that of United States natives, with a high incidence of heart disease and heart attacks. Nothing better indicates that the psychological makeup and emotional response to stress of an individual are only partially constitutional, and that they are modifiable by external factors.

Individuals who are born healthy may have minimal constitutional differences in their metabolic functions. However, within the range of normal metabolism, these differences are often amplified by environmental factors. For example, an obese individual is not obese simply because of a 'slow metabolism', as is often popularly believed and stated, but because of a vicious cycle of over-eating, which produces laziness because of the difficulty of moving an overweight body around, which in turn leads to more over-eating. A study of Harvard University students has shown that overweight students shun physical activity more than their peers of normal weight, while continuing to over-eat, or at least to eat as much as their more active, normal-weight colleagues.

So, while undoubtedly minor metabolic differences do

exist, those differences cannot account for the marked differences in weight of otherwise healthy individuals. And while we're on this subject, I would like to make the point that the use of thyroid hormone for weight reduction is unjustifiable and poor medical practice. Obviously the heart and the circulatory system are affected by such external modifiers of the physique, in that they allow the avoidance of physical activity, which is one of the most important determinants of cardiovascular fitness.

Anthropologists have classified individuals into three major constitutional groups, namely: slender, or ectomorphic; round, or fat, or endomorphic; and muscular, or mesomorphic. (There are transitions and combinations among the three groups, called meso-ecto, endo-meso, etc.) Attempts have been made to determine whether heart disease is more frequent in any of these constitutional groups. It was thought at one time that the muscular, or mesomorphic, body build is more often connected with coronary heart disease and heart attacks than the slender, or ectomorphic, body build, with endomorphic falling in between. However, as we have seen, body build is greatly modified by external factors, such as eating and physical activity; thus a relationship between a truly inherited constitutional body build and a tendency to heart attack is very difficult to determine. Researchers tried to get around this by making exact anthropological measurements – the calculation of ratios between height, arm span, specific bone lengths, head diameters, etc. – but no clear-cut evidence could be found that one specific constitutional characteristic is more frequently present in coronary heart disease.

One thus has to come to the conclusion that the constitution, as manifested in body build, metabolism, and emotional response, cannot be selected as a dominant determinant of normal cardiovascular function, or of a tendency to heart disease. In other words, your inherited constitution is so greatly modified by environmental, cultural, and other life-style factors that these factors overshadow it in determining the health of your heart.

There are, however, certain specific diseases, including heart and vascular diseases, that are connected with or related to certain constitutional abnormalities. One such constitutional abnormality is the very tall, slender body build, with long extremities, flat chest, and a characteristic head. It derives from an inherited connective-tissue weakness leading to valve defects in the heart, an enlargement and bulging of the aorta called aneurysm, a dislocation and floating of the eye lens because of lack of connective-tissue support, and other abnormalities. This condition is called Marfan's syndrome, and it occurs in certain families as part of an inherited growth defect. But this and other inherited abnormalities are not considered normal constitutional traits, and therefore cannot be considered as representative of the normal population.

To sum up, then, your inherited constitution is a mild to moderate determining factor of your cardiovascular function and your tendency to develop heart disease, but it can be strongly modified for better or worse by your environmental and life-style factors.

9

Your Emotions and Your Heart

Three of the strongest human motivators are the drive for self-preservation, the drive for personal recognition, and the drive for human contact such as friendship and sexual, familial, and other bonds.

Needing food and shelter above all else, primitive man's primary driving force was self-preservation. In modern terms, this drive is oriented towards the establishment of economic security to provide the essential commodities of life. Without success in this basic drive, the individual feels lost. The psychological impact of the fulfilment of this basic self-preservatory drive was recognized and analysed by the classical psychologists Freud and Adler, and they ranked it higher than the other two. However, with economic success and security comes the need for personal recognition and the forming of bonds, and the fulfilment of these two drives then becomes the basic prerequisite for the development of a stable emotional state. How do these emotional factors influence the health of your heart? And, vice versa, how does the condition of your heart influence your emotional life?

I indicated earlier that the way we respond to emotional stress depends not only on the inherited constitutional state of our nervous system, but to a large extent also on our cultural, family, and religious background. Taking overall American cultural and family background as a basis, it is interesting and perhaps revealing to analyse how the three basic human drives influence our emotional life.

In our culture, economic success has been, and is, one of the most important prerequisites of recognition. Striving for better, higher, and particularly for 'more' is so ingrained in us that in many instances the drive becomes a goal in itself, irrespective of what it actually produces in terms of recognition or material gain. In other words, we are emotionally wrapped up in seeking 'success' for the sake of success, irrespective of whether or not we do ourselves or others any good in the process. And, of course, such an attitude cannot but lead to many emotional tensions and psychological ups and downs. Indeed, the struggle for economic success in our complex social and economic system can and does create insecurities and anxieties which must inevitably have an impact on our physical health, in which the heart plays so critical a role.

The drive for economic success is closely tied to the drive for recognition. When the basic needs of food and shelter are fulfilled, we then immediately long for recognition, respect, and love: first from our families, then from our friends, then from our community, and sometimes even from our nation, or from the entire world. Compounding this drive is the fact that a person who is a failure may receive pity, but not recognition. A fear of failure thus fills the hearts of many, to the point where anxiety and guilt complexes develop, leading to psychosomatic illness, behavioural excesses, and addictions. I have seen patients suffering from attacks of racing or irregular heartbeat, and fear of heart attack, who in the quiet and trusting atmosphere of the surgery revealed a deep-seated anxiety and fear of failure or rejection as a causal factor. This happens because our emotional life is so closely tied in with our bodily functions through our autonomic nervous system that each one must always affect the other.

The third basic human drive is to form relationships and bonds, and it is, of course, the direct result of the first two in that a successful and respected individual will attract friends, will be able to create human ties, will be a fine lover, or whatever. Success in economic life is thus closely related to success in social advancement, in friendships, and even in the marital bed. Indeed, as all doctors know, rejection and failure in sexual life, or even in forming of lesser human bonds, can result in all kinds of psychosomatic symptoms, including cardiovascular complaints. The reason is, of course, that failure in these areas powerfully threatens an individual's basic self-respect, and therefore ultimately his survival.

The existence of these basic human drives, and their amplification by our cultural background, explains why Friedman and Rosenman found such an excessively large number of aggressive Type A people in the United States. This emotional behavioural makeup is a product of our time and our culture: we breed individuals who to thrive must succeed in all the above three areas in any and all circumstances. And, of course, such people inevitably produce more adrenalin, harbour more repressed hate, and accumulate more anxieties than the more stoic people of the Eastern cultures, where 'success' is measured differently.

But this is not to say that the aggressive Type A behavioural characteristic is necessarily in itself a primary risk factor of heart disease. Where the risks lie are in the excesses that are bred by this type of behaviour. Examples can be seen all around us daily. Watch a young executive gulp down martinis at a business-oriented social function, perhaps against his better judgement, simply because by relieving his inhibitions they allow him to be more aggressive, or witty, or 'with it', in the eyes of his superiors and colleagues. Similarly, excessive smoking, coffee-drinking, and eating are often the result of aggressive behaviour born of the need to cover up anxiety and frustration. The basic emotional need for recognition and acceptance may be fulfilled by such behaviour, but too often the price is disastrously high in terms of physical health.

A classic – and particularly sad – example of such behavioural characteristics can be seen in our teenagers. How often does it appear to you that a young person starts to smoke at an early age, not because he particularly likes it, but rather because he wants to be *accepted* – wants to be one of the crowd? No arguments about health and no reference to later physical consequences can change such youths. The only important thing is the present; acceptance and status *now*. And that – like all these emotional risk factors – is, of course, not a medical problem, but a social and cultural problem.

To sum up, our emotions are intricately tied to our cardiovascular system because of their determination of our behaviour: of how we eat, drink, smoke, work, rest, exercise, and generally live our lives. And it is in these fields that they create the risk factors, not in and of themselves as emotions.

10

Your Environment and Your Heart

Your environment is in the largest sense the world you live in: all the physical characteristics that surround you and your family and friends and community and colleagues, and your and their social, cultural, and vocational activities.

Physical environment has a great modifying effect on most people's life-style because the climate, altitude, and vegetation in which they live will basically determine their food, their work, and the activities that comprise their lives. Indeed, some of the major national and racial characteristics of the world derive largely from differences in physical environment.

Climate is thus a major environmental factor. Does it influence our heart and our susceptibility to heart disease? Except for the two extremes of equatorial heat and polar cold, only to a moderate extent is it a factor so far as presently determined by research. For example, Italians and Greeks living in Mediterranean areas have less coronary heart disease than Norwegians, Swedes, Finns, and North Americans, partly because the climate in which they live enables them to eat certain foods which grow more easily in their environment than in colder climates. Also, people living in cool or temperate countries tend to consume more animal products, particularly fats, than people living in warmer or tropical climates, who tend to consume fewer animal products and fats but more vegetable products. One reason for this, at least in the past, was that northern people, by having to perform more vigorous physical work for a living, burned up the larger amount of calories ingested in animal fats. Nowadays, however, modern transport and work-saving gadgets have largely reduced physical effort, but the eating habits suited to the old environment have not changed. This is probably one reason for the greater increase in coronary heart disease among people living in the temperate and cooler areas of the globe as compared with those of the warmer areas.

Rheumatic heart disease was found in the past to be more frequent in the temperate and colder areas, because infections spread more easily during cold weather through people congregating in crowded, heated quarters. But this difference seems to have disappeared with the treatment of streptococcal infections with antibiotics.

Climate has other implications, particularly for people who already have heart diseases. Hot, humid weather is not good for people with defective hearts and a tendency to heart failure, because it can aggravate the condition by increasing the workload on the cardiovascular system. A healthy heart, however, can stand hot, humid weather quite well provided that proper precautions are taken to permit perspiration and to prevent heat prostration or heat stroke. In hot and humid weather one cannot work as hard without running the risk of heat stroke, which obviously will affect the cardiovascular system.

These are, of course, extremes, and the question remains: Does our normal environment affect our heart and vascular system? For instance, what effect does city air pollution have on the cardiovascular system, and does it promote cardiovascular disease?

Unfortunately, the answers are not simple. City air pollution is caused more by the burning of petrol in cars, which produces carbon monoxide, than by industrial or other polluting factors. To this is added sulphur dioxide, ammonia, and carbon dioxide from burning coal and oil. The city dweller who is exposed daily to such pollutants is aware of them as an irritant to his respiratory system, particularly at higher concentrations in stagnant air, and there is no doubt that such pollutants can aggravate any existing respiratory and/or cardiovascular problems. However, there is at present no convincing evidence that pollution is directly responsible for the development of either lung cancer or coronary heart disease. It should be added here that in cigarette smoking much higher concentrations of pollutants – namely, tar products and carbon monoxide – are directly inhaled than exist in any city air pollution, and that cigarette smoking has definitely been linked with the increased incidence of lung cancer.

Environmentalists and doctors are constantly studying the question of whether or not carbon monoxide in the air of our cities is sufficiently high to affect our hearts adversely, and we are beginning to suspect that chronic exposure to it is more harmful than previously thought. In cigarette smoke the concentration of carbon monoxide is several times higher than in city air, but on the other hand the exposure of smoking is intermittent, whereas exposure to city air – particularly of those whose jobs keep them outdoors – is more continuous.

Studies have indicated that there are signs of increased carbon monoxide concentrations in people exposed to heavy car traffic, but again there is no apparent ill effect. A forty-a-day cigarette smoker has even more definite signs of chronic increase of carbon monoxide haemoglobin in his blood, yet again without apparent ill effect because of compensatory mechanisms in the haemoglobin system. Thus, it is yet to be proved whether or not concentrations of carbon monoxide in the blood resulting from chronic exposure to city air adversely affect the cardiovascular system.

Is it possible that some other effect of carbon monoxide is damaging to the body? We indicated earlier that the possibility exists that a mechanism other than hypoxia (low oxygen-carrying capacity of the blood) is responsible for the increase of chronic atherosclerosis and coronary heart disease in individuals exposed to carbon monoxide. Larger amounts of cholesterol entering the arterial wall through the slightly poisoned cells of the inner lining of the blood vessels has been suggested as a possible cause. However, much more research is needed before this mechanism can be confirmed. If it is, it will probably be found to play a much higher role in heavy cigarette smokers than in non-smokers exposed to city air pollution.

11

Your Work and Your Heart

Much has been said about work and the heart in previous chapters, so my intent here is to summarize and put into perspective how your work affects your heart and how it may contribute to your risk of developing heart disease.

Your workplace is the part of your environment where you spend a considerable, if not the greatest, part of your time. There are 168 hours in a week, so if you sleep 8 hours a night you are left with 112 waking hours. If you work 40 of these a week, counting an hour of travel each day, you are left with 67 hours a week to spend on other activities. However, many of us spend more than 40 hours a week on work, and may also travel longer to and from work, leaving perhaps no more than 50 to 60 hours per week for other activities. Since, normally, a good part of this remaining time will be spent in getting ready to go to work and at meals, it is clear that most people spend the largest single portion of their waking hours either working or in a working environment. Of course, 'workaholics' spend considerably more time at work than the average.

We pointed out earlier that the amount of daily physical activity seems to have a relationship to susceptibility to coronary heart disease, and in this respect some people perform sufficient physical activity during their work to apparently protect themselves to some degree from heart disease. However, it would seem that only a very limited number of people enjoy such protective effects for certain, in that it can be shown medically that only continuous heavy physical labour with high peaks of effort, such as those made by dock-workers and other heavy labourers, offers definite protection. Thus, while it is advisable for sedentary workers to use every opportunity to expend energy, such as walking stairs rather than using lifts, there is no evidence that such limited physical activity is protective against coronary heart disease. There is no doubt, however, that even limited exercise has the benefit of contributing to the prevention of overweight, and we will discuss this later in more detail.

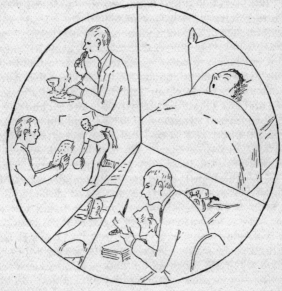

Division of time of the 24-hour day among the activities of an average businessman.

How about the emotional impact of your job? It is often implied that people succumb to heart disease as a result of psychological stress or nervous tension in their jobs, or simply from 'working too hard'. This is definitely an oversimplification. We can state categorically that *nobody* dies of hard work alone, and that other aggravating or predisposing factors have to be present in all cases of coronary heart disease. In short, emotional or stress problems at work – or even an unusually punitive physical activity – will not kill you unless you already have an underlying coronary heart disease or other cardiac problem. This is not to say, of course, that these problems will not upset you or exhaust you, especially if, as so many people do, you react compulsively to them.

Tension, emotional upsets, or excessive physical activity are in themselves only *precipitating* factors of a heart attack in the presence of an already underlying condition of coronary atherosclerosis. The real risk factors, as we've emphasized previously, are not stress or frustration in themselves, but the excesses they so often breed in modern life, namely lack of moderation in eating and drinking, heavy smoking habits, and lack of physical activity. Many men and women have encountered economic setbacks, emotional trauma, tension at work, and so on, and have been successful in performing their jobs despite all the odds, as long as their hearts were essentially healthy and their coronary arteries free of atherosclerosis. Thus, no one should overestimate the significance of work-bred tension as a risk factor in itself. Most work creates tensions and emotional ups and downs, and as long as you counterbalance these with sufficient recreation and the ability to relax and to get away from it all periodically, they will not harm you.

What about the work of the housewife? Modern technology has unquestionably decreased the amount of physical work today's housewife must perform compared with her counterpart in the past. Nevertheless, the demands and complexities of homemaking and the raising of children still keep most wives and mothers quite physically active if they take these roles seriously. If they also pursue some spare-time physical activity, rather than playing bridge or visiting over tea and biscuits, they are usually in relatively better physical shape and closer to their ideal weight than their sedentary spouses.

There are, of course, just as many frustrations and tensions in the life of a housewife as in that of her business executive husband, even though they may be of a different nature. Try, if you don't believe me, to get a plumber when your toilet suddenly overflows or an electrician when your oven burns out on the night of a dinner party; or rush a child to the hospital when he gashes his foot in the local swimming pool, then be all sweet and smiling when your tired and frustrated spouse arrives home. But, as with business stress, these things are simply a part of living, and in and of themselves they will not damage your heart. They only become risk factors when the housewife allows them to turn her frustrations into excesses or over-indulgence in eating, drinking, or smoking.

In one sense, work is actually good for your heart in that it is a great pacifier. Imagine what would happen to many people if the working week were to be shortened to, say, 20 hours. The great majority would simply not know what to do with themselves, and many as a result would become even more self-indulgent in terms of physical idleness and eating and drinking. Thus it can fairly be said that steady, creative, satisfying work, interspersed with wholesome leisure activities and exercise, and moderation in food and drink, is actually one of the best assurances of maintaining a healthy heart.

12

Your Food and Your Heart

The food you eat will affect your overall health, and it will also either protect or damage your heart.

The important ingredients in a balanced diet are proteins, carbohydrates, fats, cholesterol, minerals, vitamins, and water, and nutritionists have now established minimum recommended amounts of most of these ingredients.

Carbohydrates are contained in grains, in some vegetables, and in fruits. They are predominantly energy sources that are quickly used by your body, and the amount you need depends on your energy expenditure (or burning of calories) with each activity you undertake.

Fats are also energy sources, but they are additionally carriers of important metabolic regulators, including certain vitamins, lecithin, cholesterol, and so on. The heart muscle, for instance, uses mostly fatty acids as its energy source, and these are derived from food fats after metabolic breakdown of the fat molecule.

Proteins are predominantly body-cell builders used during the growing period, and for replacing deteriorated cells. Protein can also be used as an energy source, and in a starving person body proteins will be converted to carbohydrates to be burned as an energy source. This is the reason why people who have to perform heavy work with very little food, like prisoners of war, suffer from muscle wasting – they burn up the proteins of their muscles as their energy source. In normal circumstances, however, protein is not used by the body as an energy source.

Minerals, trace metals, and vitamins are needed for certain phases in the metabolic functions of the body, and

YOUR FOOD AND YOUR HEART 111

the minimum needed amount for most of these has been scientifically established and can be read on the labels on multivitamin and mineral preparations.

Our ancestors selected their foods by instinct and taste, not really knowing which ingredients were important or what the ingredients did to their bodily functions. At times, often because of shortages or cultural customs, their diet became somewhat unbalanced, although usually remaining simple in nature. Periodically, as a result, nutritional insufficiency developed in some areas of the world, and still does exist in several countries today. However, as the science of nutrition has developed to the point where nutritionists have been able to determine the ingredients in foods necessary for normal healthy bodily functions, the concept of the balanced diet has been established, and is now available to everyone in the Western world.

Nutritional principles are now being taught in some schools and colleges and, as eating habits are established early in life, these are very commendable programmes. It cannot be said, however, that such efforts have been successful with our population as a whole. Had they been, then the tremendous rate of new coronary heart and vascular diseases each year would not persist. Recent reports have shown a slight decrease in the rate of new coronary heart diseases, which may be an indicator that all the efforts to educate the public about nutrition are at last having some effect. However, the decrease is very small and a great deal more remains to be done before we reach, for instance, the low yearly incidence of new heart and vascular diseases of the native Japanese.

What is the problem with our nutritional education? Is what we teach inaccurate, or are we not following what we are teaching? The answer is both, to a certain degree. We teach that our diet should be 'balanced', by which we mean that it should contain all the important ingredients such as proteins, carbohydrates, fats, vitamins, and minerals. But we say very little about the *amount* of calories needed for any given amount of energy expenditure, or about the optimum distribution of calories among proteins, fats, and carbohydrates. Our youth is taught in school to seek all the essential ingredients in their food, and then after school we take them to a fast-food establishment to consume large and perhaps unnecessary amounts of protein and fats by adding a large milk-shake to a double cheese-burger with chips. And, of course, we do the same sort of thing in our homes.

The problem is not so much that our meals are not balanced, or lacking in proteins, fats, and carbohydrates, but that they are consistently *excessive* in one or more of these ingredients.

For example, protein is predominantly a building stone for cell replacement and cell growth. It has been established that after the necessary minimum amount is consumed, any excess – given sufficient carbohydrates and fats for energy – is not used by the body, but has to be detoxicated by the liver and eliminated as urea nitrogen in the urine. How much protein is necessary in our daily diet? Nutritionists tell us that a normal healthy adult needs about 40 grams daily. Ideally, half of this can be obtained from vegetable proteins and the other half from animal proteins, or from vegetable proteins which contain certain essential amino acids. Now, 20 grams of animal protein is contained in 100 grams of lean meat – or less than a 4-ounce steak. Thus a very small steak contains all the animal protein you need each day, even if you do not consume other animal protein such as milk, cheese, or eggs. The fact is, of course, that most of us eat far more protein than that each day, the excess being so much waste.

However, the greatest problem in terms of the heart is that, along with the excess protein, we are also consuming extra animal fat, because protein and fat are present to-gether in all foods of animal origin. Even the leanest meat has at least 15 per cent fat, and milk products such as cheese have a considerably greater proportion of fats. We explained earlier that animal fats are usually saturated or hard fats, and that an excessive amount of them promotes atherosclerosis by raising the blood cholesterol. So the problem is not that animal protein and animal fat are 'bad' in and of themselves, but that we *consume too much of them* by making them the main object of our culinary enjoyment. If this is true, then obviously the concept of a balanced diet has to be extended to provide us with an *optimum* rather than an excessive ratio of animal proteins, fats, and carbohydrates, along with the other essential ingredients in our food.

Since it appears that as a nation we are consuming too much of certain food ingredients, and probably too little of others, while in many cases eating an excessive number of calories in relation to our physical activity, is the problem lack of education regarding balanced nutrition, or is it that we ignore the information that we have? As with everything else in human behaviour, there can be no black and white answer.

It has become our habit to build our main meals around some animal protein product, usually meat. Grains or vegetables are often viewed largely as a sort of decoration. This type of eating is quite simply the traditional and habitual nutritional pattern of the Western world. It is usually followed at least twice a day, often after a couple of eggs and bacon or other meat in the morning. Vegetable proteins, vegetable oils, and even carbohydrates come a long way down the list in this type of eating. The problem is further compounded by the fact that most working people eat at least one meal away from home each day, and that our food and restaurant industry is geared towards satisfying the popular taste for animal protein and fat. Now add to these factors the relative physical inactivity of the nation and it is easy to see why the British population is overweight, and why its cholesterol levels are so high, and why it suffers so catastrophically from atherosclerosis.

How you can modify your eating habit for a more balanced and healthier distribution of protein, fat, and carbohydrate intake will be detailed later in this book.

What about carbohydrates, minerals, and vitamins? Even here we have adopted a number of habits which seem to be contrary to some sound nutritional principles. Instead of consuming carbohydrates from vegetables, grains, and fruits – in other words, in their most natural form – we consume relatively large amounts of artificial sugars in the form of manufactured sweets and desserts. Obesity is one result, and another is insufficiency of certain essential trace metals, such as chromium, selenium, and zinc, that are present particularly in unrefined grain, and that conceivably have an important role in protecting against heart disease. Sugars and refined carbohydrates eliminate the source of these important trace metals in our food. Then there are other trace metals which are even more important, such as magnesium, to be found in the green, leafy vegetables. Although we don't know yet whether or not a relative deficiency of magnesium has any relationship to the development of atherosclerosis, we do know that it has a role in cholesterol metabolism.

Finally, what about vitamins? Well, there is currently a great controversy about some of them, particularly vitamins C and E, in relationship to atherosclerosis and heart disease. For example, it has recently been claimed that vitamin C has an important function in the metabolism of the cells of the vascular walls. This belief holds that, when high doses of vitamin C are consumed, cholesterol trapped in the vascular wall during the process of filtration may re-enter the blood circulation and be eliminated, thus clearing the wall of cholesterol. If this is true, it would be wonderful news, since atherosclerosis could then be treated by a pill. However, critical evaluation of this effect has not as yet confirmed the claim, and, in the meantime, one has to warn against consumption of excessive amounts of vitamin C because of the possible side effects that could result, such as the formation of kidney stones.

What about vitamin E, at present consumed by some people in large amounts in supplements? We have no convincing evidence that large amounts of vitamin E intake have any beneficial effect on the efficiency of the heart muscle, or on coronary heart disease in general. Certainly no definite protective effect against atherosclerosis has been shown. A small amount of vitamin E is probably utilized by the body in its metabolic processes, but then vitamin E is present, probably in sufficient amounts for that, in the oil of wheat germ and in yellow leafy vegetables. All we can safely say about this vitamin is that gulping it in thousands of units per day may neither help nor harm your heart, but that the practice will certainly lighten your wallet.

13

Your Drink and Your Heart

Sixty-five per cent of the human body is composed of water. This water is present inside the tissue cells, between the cells in the connective tissues, and in the different body fluids, such as the blood, which transport nutrients to the cells of the different organs and also transport your metabolic by-products to the excreting organs for elimination.

The water in your body is continuously removed in some form or another, and replenished by the water you consume. The amount of water you need during any given day depends under normal conditions on the rate of your metabolism, the physical activity you perform, and your eliminatory rate by perspiration or other means. Your fluid intake is regulated by your thirst mechanism, which quite accurately indicates to you when water replacement is needed. The average amount of water consumed in different ways, such as in coffee, juices, soups, solid foods, and water itself, varies markedly but is approximately two to three quarts per day with moderate activity.

What about the water you drink? We are told in health classes that we should drink two to three glasses of water when we get up in the morning. However, many of us do not like the taste of our water, because of strong chlorination or other not so pleasant tastes, so we usually drink only juices and coffee or tea in the morning. Coffee and tea, with their caffeine and theophylline content, have a diuretic effect that leads to elimination of ingested water somewhat faster than usual. This has to be replaced by drinking water or other fluids which have no diuretic effect. Thus it is a good practice to drink several glasses of water during the course of the day.

We mentioned earlier that the practice of using 'soft water' to make washing and cleaning easier may not be beneficial in health terms. Soft water (especially when artificially softened) has a higher concentration of sodium, and the extra sodium may be a factor in causing or aggravating high blood pressure. Soft water may also dissolve from lead plumbing larger than desirable amounts of trace metals such as cadmium, which has been implicated as a possible factor in the development of high blood pressure.

Studies in the past few years in different parts of the world have shown that natives using hard water for drinking and cooking have significantly lower incidences of high blood pressure and cardiovascular disease than natives living in areas where the water is naturally soft. This is an intriguing finding, because the factor that may be involved in protecting against high blood pressure and heart disease in hard water is not completely clear. Nevertheless, some caution may be in order for those who have artificial water softeners, perhaps to the point of recommending a separate hard water supply for drinking and cooking purposes.

The West is a society of coffee drinkers – some of us consume anything from ten to fifteen cups daily! The reasons are that coffee has a pleasant taste and is a stimulant, particularly when you cannot get going in the morning. Heavy drinking of it derives in part from its diuretic effect, which causes a large part of the water consumed to be quickly eliminated, thus creating new thirst and repeated cyclical drinking. It has been found, generally but not exclusively, that cigarette smokers drink larger amounts of coffee than non-smokers, there apparently being a cross-stimulation between the two habits, or at least a similar basis existing for the two.

Is there evidence that heavy coffee drinking is related to increased incidence of coronary heart or other cardiovascular disease? Past studies have indicated that individuals drinking six to ten or more cups of coffee per day had a higher incidence of coronary heart disease than those drinking less or none. However, later studies have not confirmed this finding. Because excessive coffee drinking was often accompanied by heavy cigarette smoking, the effect of the two on the development of coronary heart disease could not be separated. Since we know that smoking has a definite bearing on coronary heart disease, it is likely that the apparent effect of coffee drinking on the development of such disease is really the effect of the accompanying cigarette smoking.

Irrespective of its effect on the heart, excess coffee drinking may have other adverse effects on the nervous system. People who are particularly sensitive to caffeine can develop nervous irritability from coffee drinking, and also increased stomach acid production which can contribute to the development of gastritis and ulcers. Moderation is thus always advisable in coffee, tea, and caffeine-containing soft drinks. I have seen attacks of anxiety and heart palpitation in individuals who were otherwise healthy but were drinking large amounts of caffeine-containing drinks, and invariably the attacks have subsided after discontinuing the practice. Even otherwise relatively calm children sometimes show hyperactivity reaction when drinking caffeine-containing soft drinks.

It would seem today that almost everyone in the Western world has at least an occasional alcoholic drink. Is there a relationship between such social or occasional (as opposed to alcoholic) drinking and heart disease, and where would the safe limits be set?

We have already alluded to the fact that what is accepted socially and by individuals as 'safe' drinking may be quite different from what is medically sound, in discussing the apparent relationship between regular pre-dinner cocktails and the body's handling of fats after a meal. Among those who like to eat foods relatively high in animal fat content, the effect of alcohol on fat absorption and the metabolism generally is even more important. As we have explained, the problem seems to be the frequency of drinking before and during meals, and the concentration of the alcohol consumed, rather than the question of whether one should or should not drink at all. The occasional social drinker who is watching both the number and size of his drinks *and* his animal fat intake does not seem to be harmed in any way. On the other hand, it would seem that the person who habitually consumes two to three drinks before every dinner, and maybe one or two before lunch, is definitely running a risk in terms of the effect on his heart through the effect on his fat and cholesterol metabolism, especially if his food preferences are high in animal fats.

When we discussed cholesterol metabolism earlier in the book, we described how alcohol raises the blood fat (triglyceride) concentration by delaying the clearing of fats from the blood. Because of this process, drinking on a continuous basis, in concert with a relatively high animal fat intake, will unquestionably promote the development of high blood cholesterol levels, and thus of atherosclerosis. Since this particular effect of alcohol depends on its concentration in the blood, the European custom of drinking small amounts of wine with meals, without having drunk highly concentrated cocktails previously, obviously leads to less amounts of alcohol in the blood, and thus to less effect on fat metabolism.

Obviously, the common sense answer is, as in so many other things, moderation. In this way will be avoided not only another risk factor in heart disease, but the psychological dependence on drinking that is the beginning of alcoholism. Frequently, this dependence starts in a subtle form with no outwardly recognizable signs, and any sensible individual who recognizes the beginnings of dependency should do his best not to drink at all. And, should he or she achieve abstinence, one thing is for certain in terms of the heart: it will certainly not be damaged by the absence of liquor.

14

Your Sleep and Your Heart

The human body is built to function in a cyclical pattern, with distinct day and night cycles. It is the central nervous system that requires 'recharging' by a period of sleep.

The amount of sleep required varies with individuals, depending upon the depth of the sleep and the regenerative power obtained from it. Some people need amazingly little sleep, only five to six hours a night throughout their lives, because they sleep so soundly and restfully that they obtain complete recharging of their nervous energy in that comparatively short period. However, most adults need seven to eight hours of sleep a night, and children and older people may need even more. Awakening tired even after a lengthy sleep happens because the sleep is restless and superficial. A frequent complaint in the doctor's surgery is, 'I sleep for nine hours or more, and awake so tired in the morning that I am hardly able to start my day.' Such complaints are the result of a lack of deep, refreshing sleep.

There are several causes of restless sleep. If the individual is physically healthy, it can be caused by insufficient physical activity during the day, combined possibly with excessive amounts of stimulants such as coffee and tea. After awakening, the individual has the feeling of not having slept at all. This then becomes a vicious circle, because by the time the poor sleeper finally begins to get going during the day, the next night cycle is upon him at a time when his nervous system is not properly conditioned for sleep. Such individuals would be much better off sleeping fewer hours and using the extra time to obtain more physical activity and recreation. Often they sleep a lot better on holiday, after hiking, swimming, or some vigorous physical activity. They would do so the rest of the time if they were simply to increase their exercise.

Exercise has the additional benefit of helping to control weight. We have shown that overweight is usually the result of excess calories, leading to decreased physical activity, and thus to even more weight gain. When this is further compounded by attempting to sleep more, physical activity is even further decreased and the weight goes up even more, further cementing the vicious circle.

The problem of not being able to fall asleep, or awaking very early in the morning after a short period of sleep, has to be approached differently. Inability to mentally 'unwind' may result in a person not being able to fall asleep, and is largely responsible for the excessive and unnecessary use of sleeping pills in Britain. Persistent inability to sleep, and particularly early awakening, requires medical attention because it may be symptomatic of other nervous problems.

While the majority of people sleep during the night, the human nervous system can adapt to a different waking–sleeping cycle without apparent harm. This happens in the case of shift workers, entertainers, and many others who must work at night. However, a certain amount of exposure to daylight seems to be necessary to good health in every human being.

15

Your Sex Life and Your Heart

Sexual drive is hormonally regulated in all living creatures for procreation and the survival of the species. In human beings, however, the natural or hormonal drive became submissive to higher nervous system control, and is today governed largely by moral, religious, social, and cultural value judgements.

We have noted that one of the strongest human drives is to form bonds, and the most important of these is the heterosexual marital bond for companionship and procreation. However, the complex interrelationship of physical sexual needs, the psychological need of companionship, and the moral, religious, social, and cultural customs of Western civilization make the sexual life of most individuals a very delicate emotional process. Much unhappiness and emotional disturbance are created by sexual misunderstanding and selfishness, and the 'sexual revolution' of recent times, plus the women's liberation movement, have further confused an already intensely complex area of life. Understanding one's own feelings in the process of seeking fulfilment of one's sexual needs is today no easy task, especially for young people.

Sexual companionship is one of the most basic human needs, and a vitally important factor in emotional stability. With all the treatises now published, scientific and otherwise, there is no need here to go into the physical aspects of sexual practices. However, as few of these books seem to pay much attention to the long-term emotional consequences of sexual contact, it might be productive to look briefly at these.

The modern sexual revolution has led to a general increase of casual physical relationships without development of emotional ties or, sometimes, even mutual respect and emotional attraction. The sexual relationship thus often becomes a purely selfish act to satisfy a physical need. This may result in temporary physical satisfaction but in the long run it too often results in emotional emptiness. Emotional contentment and healthy psychological balance are the result of unselfish giving, not of taking. In the case of most casual sexual relationships, the latter is unquestionably present. This is why the relationship developed on the basis of mutual respect and love existing in a marital bond, where giving oneself should be the emotional motive of sexual contact, is the most likely to result in a long-term healthy emotional balance.

Unfortunately, in many marriages, because there is a lack of mutual respect, or common goals, or deep-seated love, an unselfish attitude is not the basis of the sexual relationship. This can lead to emotional conflict between the physical sexual drive and the ability to give of oneself, rather than to take, and is the cause of much unhappiness and emotional imbalance. The principle of giving oneself applies to almost all aspects of human sexual life, and is the key to how frequently a healthy couple should engage in sexual activity. Mutual respect and agreement, based on the urge to give as well as receive, are the ideal sexual regulators. Given these, healthy individuals can enjoy a happy sex life well into old age, since there is no reason for limitation by age itself.

Studies have shown that during the sex act heart rate and blood pressure increase considerably. This increase, however, does not exceed that resulting from other short physical efforts usually performed several times a day even by older people. Of course, a weak ardiocovascular system or high blood pressure should be a reason for caution, and a cause for consultation with a doctor.

In a recent study it was claimed that individuals engaging in frequent sexual activity enjoy definite protection from heart disease, because of the 'tranquillizing' effect of sexual activity. Certainly, sexual activity performed in the right psychological climate has an emotionally stabilizing and tranquillizing effect – it is a common experience that sex is one of the best 'medications' for the poor sleeper. Also, through its emotionally stabilizing effect, a healthy and fulfilling sex life contributes to the prevention of heart disease by reducing or preventing frustrations that lead to over-eating, heavy drinking, and other excesses. But here again it is the *emotional* aspects of one's sex life which count for the most, far outweighing the physical aspects.

16

Smoking and Your Heart

Tobacco smoking in the form of cigarettes has been with us on a large scale for little more than a century. The introduction of the industrial production of cigarette tobacco led eventually to the manufacture and smoking of billions of cigarettes per year. Early cigarettes were rolled by hand. Later, paper tubes were prefabricated, and finally our present-day ready-made cigarettes appeared. The habit of tobacco smoking in other forms was adopted from the American Indians and taken back to the Old World by Spanish conquerors.

Although since the beginning of smoking the use of tobacco in any form has been controversial, only since the mid 1950s and early 1960s have systematic scientific studies been made on smoking and health. They have shown that 60 to 75 per cent of future adult smokers have begun cigarette smoking by the age of 18. Often the first experience with smoking occurs in primary school, and a considerable percentage of students are already habitual smokers by the time they leave secondary school. It has also been found that among the factors that promote the acquisition of the habit are parental or older sibling smoking, smoking by peers, low academic performance in school, low level of participation in school activities, low social class of family, and certain attitudes and beliefs reflecting ignorance.

Smoking is thus a *learned* habit, and one that, unlike eating and drinking, satisfies a psychological rather than a physical need. However, in some individuals the habit becomes so strong that the craving often gives the feeling of a physiological need, such as hunger or thirst. In most cases the habit is adopted early in life, and once it has been developed there are multiple reasons why it persists.

If you are a smoker, and especially a cigarette smoker, it is a certainty that you have wondered at one time or another about the harmful effects of the habit. You will then have either ignored the warnings or disbelieved the findings that support those warnings, or simply not been able to bring yourself to stop smoking even though you may intellectually recognize that it is dangerous to your health. If by some remote chance you have not recognized that already, then I must tell you that the evidence is overwhelming that cigarette smoking damages your heart, your vascular system, and your lungs. It would thus be good for you to at least fully understand *why* you continue to smoke, assuming that you do.

Studies by behavioural psychologists have shown that people smoke for different reasons; that a person may smoke for more than one reason; and that the condition initiating the smoking habit may have nothing to do with why a person continues to smoke. An individual may start smoking because of social pressure – such as teenagers experience in their desire to be 'accepted' and to demonstrate that they are growing up and conforming, etc. – but that entirely different needs or satisfactions are responsible for sustaining the smoking habit. As a result, psychologists have classified smoking from different aspects, two of which are mostly quoted in scientific literature. The first of these classifications are the need factors, such as *inner need factors* and *social need factors*.

The inner need factors characterize people who smoke because of nervous irritation: in other words, when they are 'anxious', 'irritable', 'worried', 'angry', or 'nervous'. Others in this group smoke because they want *to relax*: in other words, when they are happy, or resting after some activity, or reading or watching television. The third type in this group smoke mostly for *companionship*: in other words, their cigarettes help them to overcome loneliness (these are often individuals with heavy addiction to cigarette smoking). The fourth type in the group smoke mostly to *accompany some activity*; in other words, when they are working hard, or doing something particularly interesting, in order to help them concentrate. The fifth type uses smoking for *substitution*: in other words, to help to prevent eating in order to keep slim, or to overcome a craving for sweets.

The social factors characterize those who most likely smoke *in company*: for example, at a party, or when drinking tea or coffee, or when out for an evening. Such individuals usually smoke more during the weekend than during the week. Another social factor is the *social confidence effect* of smoking: in other words, to raise the self-confidence, to feel more sure of oneself, to feel more relaxed, to do something with one's hands when with other people.

Yet another classification has been made by analysing whether or not smokers are more likely to smoke immediately after solving a problem for a self-reward; or to get a lift during boredom; or simply for the love of smoking itself, as, for example, after meals. This is called the *positive affect of smoking*, meaning that smoking is creating a pleasant feeling or substituting for the lack of one. The *negative affect of smoking*, on the other hand, characterizes those individuals who smoke in response to unpleasant experiences, such as anger, fear, or some sort of distress. Such people may smoke heavily during a distressful day, but hardly at all when they are relaxed, or on vacation, or when enjoying pleasant experiences. While a combination of many of these factors may exist in most smokers, true psychological addiction is mostly related to negative affect experiences.

Addictive smoking is related to the fear of not having the recourse to cope with any negative affect without the availability of tobacco. Thus addictive smokers usually supply themselves with sufficient cigarettes to be certain of not running out, against the fear of cigarettes becoming unavailable at nights, or on weekends, or in remote places, etc. If they have ever experienced being out of cigarettes when they feel the need of them, they are determined that this will never happen again. Although this type of addiction is predominantly psychological, missing smoking for a comparatively extended period of time may create some physiological disturbances, such as extreme irritability, excess stomach acid production, and low blood sugar.

It will not help our main purpose to give a complete account at this point of all behavioural and psychological reasons and theories why you continue to smoke if you are a smoker. The table on pages 130 to 132 shows you how you can mark yourself on the psychological scale, and how you *can* stop smoking when you understand exactly why you should.

The physiological effects of smoking are more easily analysable than the psychological causes of the habit, although even these are not yet completely understood in all their ramifications.

Nicotine, one of the main ingredients of tobacco smoke, is also one of the strongest poisons in nature. It is a nerve poison, the effect of which is to block transmission of impulses between certain nerve-impulse switching relays. If you were to extract the nicotine from five cigarettes each containing only a medium concentration of nicotine and swallow it, the extract could kill you within three minutes.

Nicotine inhaled in cigarette smoke in smaller concentrations has the same effect on nerve transmission. By blocking the autonomic nervous system of different organs, it creates an imbalance between stimulating and relaxing impulses. This imbalance results in constriction of the smooth muscles of the small air passages in the lungs (bronchioles), narrowing their outlets and thereby curtailing the exchange of the air in the small air sacs, called alveoli. The constriction of the smooth muscles of the small blood vessels leads to increased resistance to blood flow and to increased blood pressure. Imbalance in the nerve-impulse supply to the heart itself leads to increased heart rate.

Nicotine also has an effect on the smooth muscles of the

gut and the stomach which decreases gut function (or mobility) and thus stomach acid production. This is followed by a rebound increase of acid production after the effect of smoking is over. Another effect of nicotine is to delay after a meal the clearing of fats from the blood stream by the liver, which we discussed earlier. While all these effects are measurable, they are hardly perceived by an otherwise healthy individual. Nevertheless, all of them have been linked to the causes of lung, heart, and vascular disease.

There is, for example, unquestionable evidence that chronic bronchitis and emphysema are much more frequent in cigarette smokers than in non-smokers. The effect of nicotine on the smooth bronchiolar muscles leads to entrapment of air and distension of the small air sacs, the alveoli. In chronic cigarette smokers this occurs frequently on a long-term basis, which – with the added irritant effect of other cigarette ingredients that produce chronic bronchitis – results in the chronic obstructive lung disease commonly called emphysema. While emphysema and chronic bronchitis can also develop in non-smokers, particularly when they are exposed to dust and other irritants, the frequency of chronic obstructive lung disease in chronic smokers is 10 to 20 times higher than in non-smokers.

Whether or not the repeated acute cardiovascular effects of nicotine on heart rate and blood pressure have a relationship to the development of cardiovascular disease is less clear. However, it has been shown that, in the presence of an already existing cardiac condition, the acute effect of smoking just one cigarette may precipitate an attack of angina.

The chronic effect of nicotine on fat metabolism (the clearing factor) requires further investigation before it can be conclusively shown to play a role in the development of atherosclerosis. Theoretically, however, the increased blood fats or lipoproteins after smoking should encourage atherosclerosis.

The latest investigations indicate that chronic exposure to carbon monoxide by cigarette smokers is perhaps an even

WHY I SMOKE*

Here are some statements made by people to describe what they get out of smoking cigarettes. How *often* do you feel this way when smoking them? Circle one number for each statement.

Important: Answer every question.

	ALWAYS	FRE-QUENTLY	OCCA-SIONALLY	SELDOM	NEVER
A. I smoke cigarettes in order to keep myself from slowing down.	5	4	3	2	1
B. Handling a cigarette is part of the enjoyment of smoking it.	5	4	3	2	1
C. Smoking cigarettes is pleasant and relaxing.	5	4	3	2	1
D. I light up a cigarette when I feel angry about something.	5	4	3	2	1
E. When I have run out of cigarettes I find it almost unbearable until I can get them.	5	4	3	2	1
F. I smoke cigarettes automatically without even being aware of it.	5	4	3	2	1
G. I smoke cigarettes to stimulate me, to perk myself up.	5	4	3	2	1
H. Part of the enjoyment of smoking a cigarette comes from the steps I take to light up.	5	4	3	2	1
I. I find cigarettes pleasurable.	5	4	3	2	1

J. When I feel uncomfortable or upset about something, I light up a cigarette.	5	4	3	2	I
K. I am very much aware of the fact when I am not smoking a cigarette.	5	4	3	2	I
L. I light up a cigarette without realizing I still have one burning in the ashtray.	5	4	3	2	I
M. I smoke cigarettes to give me a 'lift'.	5	4	3	2	I
N. When I smoke a cigarette, part of the enjoyment is watching the smoke as I exhale it.	5	4	3	2	I
O. I want a cigarette most when I am comfortable and relaxed.	5	4	3	2	I
P. When I feel depressed or want to take my mind off cares and worries, I smoke cigarettes.	5	4	3	2	I
Q. I get a real gnawing hunger for a cigarette when I haven't smoked for a while.	5	4	3	2	I
R. I've found a cigarette in my mouth and didn't remember putting it there.	5	4	3	2	I

HOW TO SCORE:

1. In the spaces on the next page, enter the numbers you have circled in response to the above questions: put the number you have circled for Question A over line A, for Question B over line B, etc.

2. Total the 3 scores on each line to get your totals. For example, the sum of your scores over lines A, G, and M gives you your score on Stimulation; lines B, H, and N gives the score on Handling, etc.

$$A + G + M = \text{I Stimulation}$$

$$B + H + N = \text{II Handling}$$

$$C + I + O = \text{III Pleasurable Relaxation}$$

$$D + J + P = \text{IV Crutch: Tension Reduction}$$

$$E + K + Q = \text{V Craving: Psychological Addiction}$$

$$F + L + R = \text{VI Habit}$$

Your score for each test above can vary from 3 to 15. A score of 3 to 7 is *low*; 8 to 10 is *moderate*; 11 to 15 is *high*.

* Adapted from the Smoker's Self-Test, National Clearinghouse for Smoking and Health, U.S. Public Health Service, DHEW.

more important factor in the development of atherosclerosis than the effects of nicotine. Carbon monoxide carried by the blood seems to encourage the entry of cholesterol into the arterial wall, although future investigation will have to determine the precise importance of this mechanism in atherosclerosis.

Carbon monoxide, however, has another significant effect. We discussed earlier how, by binding with part of the haemoglobin of the red blood cells, carbon monoxide eliminates them from oxygen transport to the tissue cells. In an individual with existing hardening and obstruction of the coronary arteries, this process can precipitate a heart attack by two mechanisms. In the first mechanism, the bone marrow compensates for the lack of oxygen-carrying capacity of the red cells by producing more red cells, thereby increasing the number of red cells circulating in the blood. This in turn increases the thickness (viscosity) of the blood, making it more difficult for the blood to flow through an obstructed artery. This in turn enhances clotting. In the second mechanism, the relative lack of oxygen in the presence of compromised blood flow further increases the oxygen hunger of the heart muscle.

As precipitating factors of acute heart attack, these mechanisms have to be separated from the question of whether or not carbon monoxide promotes the *development* of pre-existing atherosclerosis. However, since existing evidence indicates that coronary heart disease is definitely more frequent in cigarette smokers, future research will unquestionably determine which one – nicotine or carbon monoxide – is predominantly responsible for the development of atherosclerosis, or whether they are equally responsible, or whether some other factor is partly or jointly to blame.

If you are a smoker you have probably become conscious of the tar content of cigarettes since the rating of each brand of cigarette in the Government table of tar content is shown in cigarette advertising. Tar is a combination of several organic and inorganic chemical substances, the most significant of which is benz-o-pyrene. Benz-o-pyrene is a strongly carcinogenic chemical that is generally thought to be responsible for the increased incidence of lung cancer in chronic cigarette smokers. Also, cancer of the tongue, lips, oesophagus, stomach, and bladder in users of tobacco in other forms than cigarettes has been linked to this substance. It is not known for sure whether benz-o-pyrene is responsible for the development of atherosclerosis and heart and vascular disease, but it appears to be unlikely.

The role in atherosclerosis of most of the other chemical substances found in tobacco smoke, such as trace metals and the recently discovered radioactive materials, is not known and has not been investigated to any large extent at the present time.

The message in all the foregoing is, of course, crystal clear: smoking damages your body, and particularly your heart, vascular system, and lungs. By smoking you expose yourself to a whole host of pollutant chemicals which usually do not burden non-smokers – at least, rarely in the high concentrations and with the regularity that they burden the smoker. Public health officials and others today make great efforts to cleanse our environment of harmful and poisonous substances – sometimes with a greater fuss than we can easily understand. Yet the smoker continually and repeatedly exposes him- or herself to air pollution in a much higher concentration than exists in the worst industrial city air.

Why does this habit persist? Perhaps the root reason is the same as that which is responsible for so many other habits and life-styles that promote heart and circulatory disease. The acute adverse effects of smoking are barely perceivable by the individual, and the chronic effects are subtle before they manifest themselves in serious illness. It is only too easy to bury one's head in the sand, or to grab at any straw which seemingly appears to disprove the harmfulness of smoking.

17

Exercise and Your Heart

EXERCISE HABITS

In no other aspect has civilization affected our way of life more than in our daily physical activity.

In ancient times it was the privilege of only relatively few rich people to be attended by servants, and to be carried about. Today, almost all of us are served by machines and have our own personal transport, and these labour-saving devices multiply daily. Most of even our recent ancestors were obliged to expend considerably greater physical effort in living their daily lives than we must today. The result is that nowadays, to maintain even a relatively low level of physical fitness, most of us have to make a special effort to 'exercise' our muscles. Unfortunately, far too few of us take the trouble and time to perform sufficient daily exercise to keep ourselves reasonably fit – or even basically healthy. And this unquestionably is one area of life where the past really was the 'good old days', in that exercise then was a matter of necessity simply to survive, rather than choice for the sake of good health.

Exercise has many beneficial effects. Primary among them are the sense of well-being deriving from the resulting physical fitness, the calming of the nervous tension which all of us have to face daily, the maintenance of ideal weight, and the diminution of the risk of developing heart and circulatory disease.

There are several misconceptions regarding exercise, and the first one that should be cleared up is that obesity is solely the result of over-eating. The food we eat provides the calories for our bodily functions and daily activities. Whenever we do not use up all the calories we eat, the excess is deposited as fat. Therefore, overweight is the result of *unused calories due to low levels of energy expenditure* just as much as it is the result of eating too many calories. This is why many obese people claim that, even when they eat very little, they still gain weight. Much obesity, as we explained earlier, arises from a vicious cycle of 'weight gain – less physical activity – more weight gain.'

Some people refuse to exercise because they have the misconception that the effort needed for more physical activity will not increase their calorie expenditure sufficiently to reduce their weight. Some also believe that their appetite will increase with exercise, resulting in an even greater food intake that will more than make up for the extra energy expenditure and thus keep them overweight. Both of these beliefs are erroneous. It has been shown that regular increase of energy expenditure at a moderate level can actually decrease calorie intake by suppressing the appetite. For instance, 100 calories of energy are expended by 19 minutes of brisk walking or ten minutes of jogging (see tables in Appendix I). Therefore, a loss of 25 pounds in a little over four months can be achieved by lowering the daily caloric intake by 400 calories, combined with 30 minutes of daily brisk walking.

Let us consider how many calories you usually expend per day if you are, say, an office worker, weigh 155 pounds, have a mostly sedentary job, and move and walk around to some extent during the day but have no particular exercise programme and do very little around the house after work. If you sleep eight hours, you consume 560 calories during the night (you expend 70 calories per hour during sleep). In getting ready for work, and being at ease during the work period for say a total of two hours per day, you expend 250 calories. Let's say you walk to and from your car, at home and in the car park, and walk around at work for about an hour: that's 150 calories. Driving your car or travelling by train to and from work for half an hour each way burns another 100–150 calories. Working at a desk for eight hours, with interruptions, discussions, and conferences, expends approximately 1,000–1,200 calories. Eating and doing light work around the house say for one hour burns 250 calories. Let's say you spend the remaining three hours out of the 24 reading or watching TV: that's 350 calories. Your total caloric expenditure during this average day is therefore approximately 2,500–2,800.

Now, if you eat only 100 calories (one slice of bread with butter) more than that each day, you will gain 10½ pounds in a year. When you learn that the average British diet provides 2,500 to 3,500 calories per day, you can see why the nation is overweight as well as Great.

Only by increased physical activity can this kind of excessive calorie intake be counterbalanced without weight gain. And since so many of us experience relatively little obligatory physical activity and energy expenditure in our daily work and life, a planned regular exercise programme would seem to be a primary requirement for the maintenance of ideal weight and thus for good health.

Regular *intense* physical activity or exercise has a number of physiological and psychological benefits. It increases your physical fitness. It improves the efficiency of your circulatory system, indicated by the reduction of your required coronary blood flow at rest and during exercise. It increases the work capacity and the efficiency of oxygen transport by your blood and the oxygen's utilization by your tissues. It decreases the resistance in the blood vessels of your musculature, thereby decreasing your arterial blood pressure. The metabolic effect of exercise can result in improved glucose tolerance, and thus less rise of blood fats and triglycerides following a meal. While it will not in itself lower your cholesterol, intense exercise does have a beneficial effect in preventing atherosclerosis by contributing to the removal of some of the cholesterol deposited in your arterial walls. It decreases the coaguability of your blood, and thereby improves your protective mechanism against blood clots. It quite possibly increases the number of communicating blood vessels in your coronary circulation, thereby improving your chance of surviving a heart attack. And its psychological effect improves your self-respect, your feeling of well-being, your tolerance of psychological stress, and – most likely – your overall life style.

Unfortunately, not all forms of exercise have these beneficial effects. To increase the blood flow through the muscles and through the heart for more or less extended periods, the exercise must be fairly strenuous. Jogging, walking briskly, swimming, and other forms of activity which rhythmically tense and relax your muscles are the exercises that will most improve your physical fitness and have the most beneficial effects on your cardiovascular system. These are called isotonic exercises.

The forms of exercise which tense muscles only to increase their strength, such as weight-lifting, do not increase the blood flow *to* the muscles, but rather squeeze the blood *out* of the muscles. Although they will certainly strengthen the muscles and increase their tone, they will not lead to significant increase in physical fitness or result in increased stamina. Thus these so-called isometric forms of exercise do not condition the cardiovascular system to the same degree as isotonic exercises.

Isotonic exercises are also called 'aerobic' exercises, because the oxygen supply of the muscles used is sustained during the period of activity. For this reason, short maximum efforts such as 100-yard sprinting are not aerobic forms of exercise because you cannot sustain the resulting high blood flow in your muscles for longer than a few seconds, instead of for minutes or hours.

We will detail later in the book the different isotonic and aerobic exercises that most people can perform most practically.

Other requirements of exercise, if it is to improve physical fitness, are that it be performed for a sufficient length of time at each session, and that the sessions be repeated a sufficient number of times. For example, a brisk walk on level ground at 3½ miles per hour for 30 minutes daily or jogging for 15 minutes five days a week will measurably improve your physical fitness. Naturally, the specific amount of exercise that will most benefit you personally has to be governed by your age, your weight, your present level of fitness, and any physical handicap you may have, which suggests that an exercise programme should be followed under medical supervision, especially at the outset.

In addition to following a formal programme, it is obviously common sense to expend energy whenever you have the opportunity during your daily life, such as walking up stairs and walking whenever possible rather than riding. This in itself will give you a certain amount of basic fitness. However, to obtain real benefits from exercise, you must regularly reach a certain level of energy expenditure.

As we explained earlier, there is a limit to the amount of blood the heart can circulate during a maximal effort (called 'maximal cardiac output'). This limits the amount of oxygen that can be delivered to the tissues to the amount of blood that can be delivered to these tissues by the heart. The maximum amount of oxygen delivered by the blood to the tissues determines the amount of oxygen you are using from the air you inhale during breathing. This is called 'maximum oxygen uptake', and also 'maximal aerobic capacity', or 'power'. It has been shown that a person has to reach 70 to 85 per cent of this maximal aerobic power during every exercise session to improve physical fitness and obtain the fullest benefits from it.

Since the increase of heart rate during exercise is proportional to the increase of cardiac output (and thus to oxygen uptake or aerobic power), one can estimate the level of exercise by counting the heart rate during exercise. This enables you to measure whether or not a desirable level of aerobic power has been reached for a given amount of exercise performed.

Naturally, the amount of exercise required to reach 70 to 85 per cent of maximum heart rate varies with individuals and depends, in addition to age, on the present state of physical fitness and health. Once a certain level of conditioning is attained, a more strenuous exercise can be performed to attain the target heart rate because of the improved oxygen delivery by the cardiovascular system. The table on page 163 shows the age-adjusted maximal heart rate and the desirable 70 to 85 per cent 'target zone' that should be reached by a healthy adult to condition the cardiovascular system effectively.

How to plan an exercise programme, the precautions you should take, and how you can measure the amount of exercise needed to improve your conditioning will be detailed in the next section.

PART THREE

*How to Keep Your
Heart Healthy*

18

How to Choose Your 'Heart-Saver' Food and Drink

Can *you* eat and drink 'heart-saving' foods and beverages and still enjoy life? Can *you* develop the *habit* of eating and drinking thus? You most certainly can.

Your present eating habits have been ingrained in you since childhood and are the result of tradition, custom, and the availability of particular foods. As an adult, your taste is thus inclined towards certain foods primarily because of habit. People's habits vary markedly around the globe. A meal which may be very tasty to you will not necessarily appeal to a Japanese in Japan, and you might not care at all for a dish people in China consider a delicacy. Your taste, however, *can* be re-trained to like foods that you have not tasted before, or have been prejudiced against because of ignorance.

When you have modified your present eating habits to a heart-saver eating habit, you will do three things: (1) change both the amount and the composition of the food ingredients you are presently consuming; (2) learn to include in your menu new food ingredients and dishes you were not accustomed to before; (3) *thoroughly enjoy your new heart-saver meals*.

I stress the third point because eating is one of life's greatest pleasures. That being the case, the goal of your heart-saver diet is to give you maximum culinary pleasure without the danger of excesses in food ingredients that promote high blood cholesterol. This almost certainly will require some re-training of your taste, but I can assure you that you will enjoy your food after adapting to the new eating habit just as much as you enjoyed food previously.

We have presented much convincing evidence that higher than desirable blood cholesterol is a major risk factor in the development of atherosclerosis and its consequences, heart attacks, strokes, and vascular disease. From this it is impossible not to conclude that, in the vast majority of people, high blood cholesterol is directly related to the high animal fat content of the traditional Western eating patterns. Modification of daily eating habit to decrease animal fat consumption substantially and substitute vegetable oils will significantly decrease the blood cholesterol level in most individuals. That will decrease their chance of developing atherosclerosis, or the progression of an already existing atherosclerotic condition. Additionally, there is evidence that early atherosclerosis regresses as a result of changing to a low animal fat eating habit.

By changing your eating habits, therefore, you decrease your risk of heart attack. By how much? Well, to answer that let's use the risk score of a 40-year-old. A change of blood cholesterol from the moderate elevation of 280 mg per 100 ml to 220 mg per 100 ml, given the absence of high blood pressure and no cigarette smoking, can decrease a 40-year-old's risk for the next 12 years from approximately 6 per cent to 3 per cent. That is *half* the risk.

In planning a heart-saver eating habit, there are a few basic rules you should learn and keep always in mind, both to help you to make the change and to help you adhere to the new habit even in difficult eating circumstances, such as travelling or staying in somebody's home. If you follow these principles, it will not be necessary literally to calculate calories, saturated and unsaturated fats, proteins, carbohydrates, etc., every time you eat. Very quickly you will learn to make intelligent and sound decisions simply by looking at the available food. And if at times you are obliged to exceed what you think is the proper limit, there is no need to panic, because you can make up for it the next or in following days by simply restricting your food intake as you feel appropriate. In the long run, the *overall* average is what counts.

Based on modern concepts of wholesome, balanced, heart-saver nutrition, these are the principles you should always keep in mind:

1. Your calorie intake always should stay in balance with your energy expenditure. If you are of 'ideal weight', you will then maintain that ideal weight. If you are above ideal weight, you should not only decrease your calorie intake but also increase your energy expenditure by increasing your physical activity.

2. Decrease the emphasis on animal fats and protein in your food by serving yourself only modest portions of meat, such as a steak the size of your palm (half an inch thick) or modest pieces of mostly white meat of chicken or turkey, etc. Even the leanest meat contains 10 to 20 per cent animal fat, so to minimize fat intake cut off all excess fat from all the meat you eat. Likewise, don't eat the skin of chicken or turkey because it contains a high proportion of fat. Eat beef or pork not more than three times a week. The rest of the time eat chicken, turkey or fish (not shellfish), all of which contain less saturated fats than the 'red' meats.

3. Grill, roast, or bake meat and fish instead of frying them. These forms of cooking will eliminate considerable amounts of fat from the meat – fat that you do not need. Likewise, do not use dripping for gravy or other purposes – discard it.

4. Cut down cholesterol intake by eating not more than three egg yolks per week, including those you eat in other foods, and shellfish (lobster, shrimps, oysters) not more than once a month. Avoid liver, kidney, and other offal – they contain large amounts of cholesterol and fats.

5. Use liquid dressings for your salad, such as vinegar and oil and Italian dressing, in preference to mayonnaise. Avoid all animal shortening and butter, using corn and sunflower

oil for cooking and soft margarines for baking and spreading. Avoid all commercial fillings and frostings or glaze, because they are prepared with animal shortening.

6. Use no cream, sweet or sour, for any purpose, and avoid all cheeses with high fat content (there are now many cheeses with low fat content). Cut down on sweets and ice cream, and reduce your use of refined sugar to a minimum. Use wholemeal flour instead of white whenever possible. Reduce white bread and roll consumption and substitute wholemeal and rye breads that have high bran content. The improved digestion that will result will keep your food and calorie intake down, and probably also decrease fat and cholesterol absorption from your gut.

7. Don't imagine that you will starve with all these restrictions. To provide the calories for your energy needs, learn to eat more vegetables, fruits, and carbohydrates from whole grains. In other words, eat whole-grain cereals, wholegrain and rye bread, brown rice ('unpolished'), beans, peas, carrots, and green-leaf vegetables (preferably mildly cooked or raw), fresh fruits (apples, pears, peaches, etc., preferably with their skins). These foods will provide all the calories you need for energy expenditure without raising your blood cholesterol, and also will have the additional beneficial effect of regulating your bowel habits. (In this respect, there is evidence that cancer of the gastrointestinal tract, particularly of the colon, may be less frequent in individuals who eat less refined foods and the greater amount of roughage that comes from the bran-containing products.)

8. Eat three regular meals each day, and *never* eat snacks between them. If you feel the need for a snack, try an apple, some raw carrots, celery, or rye biscuits – or other similar foods that will not provide you with excess fat.

9. Avoid excessive amounts of coffee, tea, and caffeine-containing soft drinks. These not only stimulate your brain, heart, and circulation, but also your stomach acid production and thus a feeling of hunger. Drink instead natural fruit juices, decaffeinated coffee, skim milk, and water.

Memorize these nine points, and you will be able to select heart-saving dishes and portions wherever you may have to eat. Doing so will become your habit and part of your second nature in no time at all, and once that happens you will have no difficulty whatsoever in maintaining these habits.

Let's illustrate more graphically the effects of different eating habits. George and Joe are going out to dine together. George is eating as he learned in his childhood and always has since then. Joe is trying to keep his blood cholesterol down and has learned how to select food accordingly in a restaurant. George chooses the following:

> Tossed salad with creamy Russian dressing
> Prime steak, medium rare (10 to 12 ounces)
> Baked potato with sour cream
> Green beans with bacon
> Roll and butter
> Chocolate sundae
> Coffee with cream

Joe's choice might seem similar in some ways, and yet it is different:

> Tossed salad with vinegar and oil dressing
> Rye biscuits without butter
> Prime steak, medium well done (6 to 8 ounces)
> Baked potato with margarine
> Pineapple water-ice (two scoops)
> Black coffee

With his meal, George consumed approximately 1,776 calories; 95 grams of protein; 77 grams of saturated fats, 70 grams of unsaturated fats and 8 grams of polyunsaturated fats for a total of 155 grams of fats; 87 grams of carbohydrates; and 565 mg of cholesterol.

Joe consumed approximately 1,135 calories; 67 grams of protein; 66 grams in total fats with 31 grams of saturated fats, 32 grams of unsaturated fats, and 4 grams of polyunsaturated fats; 75 grams of carbohydrates; and 292 mg of cholesterol.

The two men, George and Joe, ate essentially the same dinner, but chose their portions, dressings, and desserts differently. The result was that Joe consumed one third fewer calories, one third less protein, less than half the total fats and saturated fats, and about half the cholesterol that George ate. This being the main meal of the day, and assuming that Joe uses similar judgement in his other two meals and snacks, he probably consumes less than 2,500 calories a day, a comparatively low level of saturated fats, and probably less than 300 mg of cholesterol per 1,000 calories per day. On the other hand, George probably consumes more than 3,000 calories per day, including excessive amounts of protein and saturated fats, and some 500 mg or more of cholesterol per 1,000 calories per day. If they are both moderately active, Joe will maintain his ideal weight while George will gain. What is even more important, George's cholesterol will increase excessively and will become, if it is not already, a significant risk factor.

Everyone can learn to eat dishes that are extremely palatable but that are low in fats and cholesterol. It is true that initially it might take more effort and patience to try something you have never tried before. But today's nutritionists, cooks, and menu planners have developed a wide variety of excellent dishes low in animal fat and cholesterol content, many of them adapted from all over the world to suit the Western taste. These are contained in a number of excellent cookbooks, such as the British Heart Foundation cookbook,* in addition to which many newspapers and magazines now publish heart-saver menus. Some sample menus for people who want to reduce their blood cholesterol appear in an appendix to this book.

Joe, of course, has recognized that his life and future

* *Cooking to Your Heart's Content*, British Heart Foundation, 1976. Available from the British Heart Foundation, 57 Gloucester Place, London W1.

largely depend upon his way of eating and drinking, but there are many who close their eyes to this fact, and others who simply seem to lack the willpower to change their habits – even after a heart attack. I recall one man who said to me, 'Doctor, I love greasy foods and gobble up everything that I can put on my plate.' He was frustrated because he had the *desire* to change his habits, but could not do so because excessive eating had become compulsive. He would sometimes starve himself all day, then at night 'clean out the entire refrigerator', to use his own words. Then there are the compulsive eaters who deceive themselves by never eating in the presence of others, and, generally claiming to eat very little, consume large quantities of rich food in private. Such people have a psychological problem that may require the help of a behavioural psychologist, who will work on the problem in cooperation with the family doctor. Obviously in all cases the primary need is a clear understanding of why a change of eating habit is necessary, and a willingness to believe in and accept the physician's advice.

When selecting food, and especially when contemplating changes in your eating habits, there is one more point which is worth keeping in mind. We have seen that high blood pressure is a major risk factor in the development of atherosclerosis. There are believed to be two factors in eating and drinking which enhance the development of high blood pressure, one of them being overweight. It is thus important that you maintain an ideal weight – and to do so, besides decreasing your calorie intake, you will probably also have to increase your physical activity. Tables in the appendix will give you an idea of how many calories to consume, and how to select your food and drink, both to maintain your ideal weight and to lose weight. The calorie expenditure necessary with certain physical activities will be discussed later.

The other element in food which may promote high blood pressure, and which often is used to excess, is salt (sodium).

We have explained why and how excess salt may be related to the development of high blood pressure, and, in view of this, use of the salt-cellar every time you eat, often even before tasting your food, is not a good practice. Some people consume more than five to ten times the amount of sodium their body functions actually require, and this may be an important factor behind the high incidence of high blood pressure in our country. The answer is to learn to like and use other seasonings whenever possible in place of salt. There are many different, pleasant-tasting seasonings which are harmless, such as lemon juice on salad and vegetables.

If you cannot do without salt, remind yourself that most of the time it is the excesses that hurt you, and that therefore moderation is the key word.

19

How to Stop Smoking

The overwhelming evidence about the harmfulness of smoking to health generally, and particularly the evidence showing smoking to be one of the strongest risk factors in heart disease, cannot but convince you, if you are a smoker, that you should stop the habit. The harmfulness of smoking, and the multiple dangers of the different ingredients of cigarette smoke, are indisputable. If they make you want to stop, the imperative starting point is your personal decision to do so. Nobody can make this decision for you but yourself.

In making that decision, you should understand that it *is* possible for anyone to stop smoking, that hundreds of thousands have done so, and that there are different techniques and aids available to help you shake the habit. Almost certainly you will have to struggle, but it will be one of the most worthwhile efforts you've ever made in your life because of its multiple rewards. Not only can you guarantee yourself a longer and healthier life by stopping smoking, but you will discover that there are some additional and maybe some unexpected benefits. For example, food will taste much, much better (maybe too good at times!), your sense of smell will return, and you'll lose that miserable morning cough. You will be proud of your independence and willpower; happier with yourself no longer to be a slave to a habit that you might have grown to hate. You will be able to breathe again more deeply. Your stamina will increase because your lungs will not be handicapped in performing their natural function. And you will save money – quite a lot if you were a forty-a-day smoker.

People who continue to smoke in the face of the irre-futable dangers of the habit do so for many reasons, but the chief one is fear. There is fear of withdrawal symptoms; of not being able to fall back on a crutch; of being irritable and miserable with family and friends. These fears make it easy to talk yourself out of accepting the evidence about the damaging effects of smoking and the improved quality of life after stopping. You may know that your arguments are weak, but nevertheless you try to justify your indecision.

A popular excuse is a grandfather who smoked all his life and lived beyond 90 years of age. What is ignored is the fact that he might have lived that long for many other reasons, such as heavy physical activity, a simple life, and relatively moderate smoking. Another popular argument is that it's too late to stop, and what's the point anyway? – all of us have to die from something. What is ignored here is the possibility of extending life by twenty or even thirty years, or of not becoming an invalid at an age when life can still be highly active and productive. Then there's the story about eating too much and becoming overweight, which is just as dangerous. A carefully planned physical activity programme and meal planning in conjunction with the effort to stop smoking will prevent that happening.

Yet another popular argument for continuing to smoke is that there is disagreement among the experts regarding the harmfulness of the habit. Don't kid yourself. Over 60 per cent of doctors who previously smoked have stopped smoking cigarettes. They have done so because they know that the disagreements are superficial: they cannot alter all the heavily indicting scientific evidence against smoking.

Occasionally doctors will come across people who argue that they don't hurt anybody but themselves by damaging their health, and there are indeed individuals who sub-consciously are truly self-destructive. However, it is rare when such a 'don't give a damn' attitude fails to go beyond the particular individual, because we influence our environ-ment by everything we do – nobody is an island in this life.

Frequently there are children whose decision to smoke or not to smoke depends very much on the example of those around them. The same is true of friends and colleagues. And when a person becomes ill because of his or her smoking habit, does he or she not hurt loved ones and dependants?

I will never forget the heartbreaking picture of a young woman who, after one unhappy marriage, found great happiness and companionship with a charming, intelligent, and successful businessman with great human qualities. In the midst of all their happiness, this man went to his doctor because of some low back pain recently developed. He had no other symptoms and thought it was just a little sprain. All tests were negative but the pain did not respond to treatment. A bone scan was done which showed a small area possibly cancerous, and it was clear that the cancer must have been transplanted from somewhere else in the body (known as 'metastasis'). The chest X-ray was normal, but the doctor examined the sputum, which also showed some suspect cells. The bronchoscopy (visual examination of the bronchi by a small mirror) discovered a small adenocarcinoma of the lung, the most devastating and rapidly metastasizing cancer of the lung. Despite all the efforts of modern medicine, the man was dead in three months. Needless to say, he had been a forty-a-day cigarette smoker from the age of twenty until his death at age forty-four.

Adenocarcinoma of the lung is almost exclusively the result of cigarette smoking. In this case there were no symptoms or warning signs, and a life was extinguished in three months in great suffering, with a conscious mind and probably agonizing feelings of guilt. This man loved his wife and her child, but he did not love them enough to stop smoking in time. Maybe he did not know better. However, those left behind were the real sufferers of the tragedy, with a burden that they will carry the rest of their lives.

You may argue that you have tried to stop smoking, but never felt much better as a result, or were actually more miserable because of the resulting irritability. The problem here is that you almost certainly did not give your body a chance to regain its vitality by correcting so far as possible the already present damage caused by smoking. How quickly and effectively your body can restore the damaged functions depends on how long you have smoked and how many cigarettes per day you have smoked. But, whatever the length of time, you *always* will benefit from stopping smoking, even if you have advanced lung and vascular damage. The reason is that, by continuing, you will accelerate the process of damage, whereas by stopping you will decelerate it.

Thus, you can see that there are no sound reasons to support a case against stopping smoking. You should, therefore, start to think positively about the beneficial aspects of stopping – the first step in acquiring the determination to break the habit.

CONDITIONING YOURSELF TO STOP SMOKING

When you finally make your decision to stop smoking, you will almost certainly have to condition yourself for the final step, because it is never easy to overcome the initial road-blocks and early difficulties.

Smoking is an ingrained habit like, for instance, turning right at the intersection each morning on your way to work. You have learned the road so well that you could make the turn with your eyes closed, and would have to deflect your thoughts consciously from the familiar road in order to take a different direction. In the same way, you will have to learn to occupy your mind with new and different thoughts to divert it from smoking. There are numerous tricks you can use to do this – the most simple being to start consciously putting your cigarettes in a different place where they are less easily accessible. At the same time, keep a little notebook in the pocket where you have previously carried your cigarettes and make a mark in it each time you smoke a cigarette. This will remind you of the cigarettes you have smoked but actually didn't want to, and it will also give you a record of how many you smoked that day. When out of habit you reach for the pocket where you previously carried your cigarettes, you will grab the notebook, which will remind you of your decision not to smoke. The power of habit will make you reach for the pocket several times a day, and force you to go to the unaccustomed place when you want a cigarette. The resulting delay will condition you to what caused you to initiate the change in the first place – that is, stopping the habit.

Because cigarette smoking is often a negative- or positive-affect habit, you may have to learn to use substitution at times when previously you have used cigarettes. Taking out a cigarette and lighting it is often a ceremonial process. For example, you may have noticed that many people, when discussing a point and having to give an answer or decision, take out a cigarette and light it quite slowly and ceremonially. Here they are using the cigarette-lighting process to gain time to think. In much the same way smokers meeting new people and finding it difficult to start a discussion will try to gain time to think about a subject by lighting a cigarette. Thus it becomes important in stopping to find other ways to gain time.

To light and smoke a cigarette involves many parts of the body, not only the thinking process just illustrated. The hands are very active, as is the mouth in performing certain manoeuvres while puffing. The smoke is inhaled with a certain gusto, and a particular type of breathing is involved. Then again the hands come into play as the cigarette is removed from the mouth and the ashes tapped into the ash-tray. All these moves are very noticeable to non-smokers, while smokers make them subconsciously. Thus it will help in stopping to consciously make some simple substitutions for all these activities whenever the urge to smoke hits you.

You should be prepared particularly to do something with your hands. At leisure, for example, try holding and shuffling a pack of cards, or manipulating a puzzle, or even simply holding a book. To substitute for the feeling of a cigarette in your mouth, chew gum or a sweet, or nibble on a stick of carrot or celery, or even a stalk of grass. I have a friend who carried a pipe around and handled it or chewed on the stem while stopping smoking. The pipe had never been used for smoking and thus did not have the tempting taste of tobacco.

When you feel the urge to inhale, do some breathing exercises, or stretch out your chest and take several deep, slow inhalations and exhalations. Sipping slowly on a glass of iced water or fruit juice can also be very helpful at these times.

If you find it difficult to concentrate because you do not have your stimulating 'smoke', lean back in a chair, close your eyes, and say to yourself without sound: 'I am relaxed, my body, arms, and legs are relaxed. I concentrate only on being relaxed. I am completely relaxed.' Repeat this for two to three minutes, and then suddenly open your eyes and return to whatever you were doing. (We'll discuss this relaxation training later in more detail.)

Although you can't do this sort of thing in company or during business, you can achieve the same result of gaining time by carrying something like a packet of peppermints in your pocket. Take them out at critical times; unwrap them slowly, and offer them to your friends or colleagues. That way you can gain at least as much time for thinking as in going through the ceremony of lighting a cigarette.

Substitutions also help in breaking the habit of smoking at specific times or in connection with specific events – for example, the habit of lighting a cigarette after a meal, or with a cup of coffee. Many people start the day with a smoke after their morning cough starts, because they feel a cigarette helps them to awake and suppress the coughing. Obviously, this is an illusion. The thing to do when you awake is to get up quite quickly and take a refreshing shower or bath, rubbing your skin vigorously as you dry yourself. When you have finished, start a short breathing exercise by slowly taking deep breaths and exhaling as far as you can after each. Rest after the deep breathing for a few seconds by taking a few normal breaths. Then do a few arm exercises, stretching your arms up and down and to the side. Jog a few times on the spot, then quickly dress and sip a glass of water as you are preparing breakfast.

After meals, occupy your hands and mouth with some sort of substitute such as a toothpick, or chew on a carrot while you are relaxing and thinking. Try to avoid coffee breaks and the slow, relaxing drinking of coffee after meals – these moments are the most conducive to smoking, especially when others are doing so. Drinking less coffee, incidentally, will also improve your health, and as you give up smoking you'll probably find less desire for coffee, because smoking and heavy coffee drinking often go hand in hand.

If you are serious about giving up smoking, it is vital that you develop the image of a non-smoker. What you particularly don't need at this stage is the teasing of smoking acquaintances with such remarks as, 'You'll never make it,' and 'I wonder when you'll give up trying?' and 'Come on, enjoy a last one.' So avoid such people. Avoid also, at least in the beginning, bars and other locations where a lot of smoking is going on.

You have to imprint the new non-smoking image of yourself strongly in your mind before you can face the overwhelming temptations. The first step in doing that is to continually state to yourself: 'I don't smoke any more.' When you are offered a cigarette, say simply, 'Thank you, I don't smoke.' Don't apologize, explain, or feel embarrassed – not smoking is more of a virtue today than smoking. When a discussion of smoking develops, don't be defensive about your non-smoking – don't offer big explanations about the harmfulness of smoking, or tell people that you read this or that book or article, but simply say: 'I decided not to smoke because I think it's better for me.' There will always be some wise guys who know better, because smokers are sometimes like addicts who want the sense of security that comes from having everyone else hooked on their drug. But, having examined the facts and made your decision, your best defence is the simple statement: 'I don't smoke.' This will better than anything else establish your image as a non-smoker, as far as both yourself and others are concerned.

We examined earlier the reasons why people continue to smoke, and these have some bearing on the problems encountered when trying to stop. For example, positive-affect smokers usually have it easier than negative-affect smokers, because negative-affect smoking is more often a psychological dependence, or even an addiction. When that's the case it is generally more difficult to overcome the initial hurdles. But don't be discouraged. *Everybody* can give up smoking. What counts most is the *decision* to do so. Given that, as we'll now see, there are various techniques that can help you to actually do the job.

HOW TO GIVE IT UP

Once you have made your decision, you should carefully plan your strategy. You can decide to stop abruptly, in which case you will have to cope with the psychological side effects of giving up, the irritability and the craving period. ASH* can give you information on support programmes available in your area. To cope with the initial withdrawal problems, most of the programmes recommend certain activities which keep you busy and take your mind off your feeling of craving, and offer substitutions for the different aspects of smoking to which you were accustomed.

If you decide that your strategy will be a gradual decrease and an eventual tapering off to zero, there are several tricks

* Action on Smoking and Health, 27 Mortimer Street, London W1.

that might be helpful. One is to change to the brand which
you least like. Another is to ration yourself by counting out
each morning the number you have decided to smoke,
placing the rest somewhere out of easy access – decreasing
your allowance daily. Keeping your cigarettes in a different
pocket or desk drawer so that you have to make an extra
effort to get them is another helpful device. Another is to
delay reaching for a cigarette as long as possible every time
you get the urge to smoke. Yet another is to try to smoke
each cigarette only halfway and later even less.

Whichever you choose, the basic task is to sustain your
determination to decrease the number of cigarettes you
smoke each day. If your irritability increases, you should
increase your physical activity and breathing exercises to
the point where sheer tiredness helps you to overcome the
problem.

One day, if your will is strong enough, you will smoke
your last cigarette. But don't make deals with yourself delaying the day of complete stopping beyond the point of
your initial resolve. The danger of relapse is great. You need
continuing dedication to your timetable if you are really
going to break the habit. And in this respect a relatively
rapid tapering off is more effective than a very prolonged
process with repeated compromises, because that way you
can maintain the initial force of your decision and thus
shorten the difficult phase of withdrawal. In fact, it is better
not to prolong the tapering-off method beyond two weeks.

HOW TO STAY OFF SMOKING

Statistics show that almost any method of stopping smoking
has an initial success rate of around 70 to 80 per cent.
Strong initial motivation, caused usually by vigorous reali-
zation of the damaging effects of smoking, is responsible for
this high percentage. But follow-up evaluation of most
techniques after a year or so shows a drop in the number

still off cigarettes to around 20 per cent. Obviously, then, the greatest problem is maintaining the initial conviction that smoking is harmful and the determination to stay away from it that goes with such conviction.

What are the factors which make people relapse? There are several. Rationalization of the habit takes over as initial enthusiasm to stop fades away. Related habits such as social functions, alcohol drinking, business luncheons and dinners, friends and colleagues who still smoke, and lack of support from family members and others commonly set the stage for recidivism. 'One cigarette won't hurt you' is probably the most dangerous siren call, yet it is that one cigarette that can and does start the habit all over again.

It is important, therefore, that you understand and guard against these and like sources of discouragement and temptation. Continue to remind yourself of your commitment and your reasons for stopping smoking. Tell yourself, 'I choose not to smoke', indicating to yourself that it was your *conscious free will* decision not to smoke, rather than some outside force, or coercion, or mere fear. If your friends or colleagues or family members tease and test you to the point where your willpower is threatened, be frank with them and tell them that you made a definite commitment not to smoke, that it is quite difficult for you even under favourable circumstances to stay off smoking, and therefore you would greatly appreciate their help, support, and sympathy.

Initially you may want to avoid any particular social function where you know that a lot of smoking will be going on. A convivial atmosphere and smoke-filled air are unnecessary temptations until your new non-smoking determination and image are sufficiently established. If you have been accustomed to lighting a cigarette while drinking coffee, or after a meal, switch to some other beverage such as tea or fruit juice to help break the association. Getting up soon after your meal to busy yourself with other things helps to eliminate the post-meal cigarette association. In general, use substitutions for the habitual bodily functions that go with smoking.

Developing a relationship with a friend or colleague who has stopped smoking at the same time as you can be very helpful, especially if it goes to the point where you can talk to him or her or ring up when you have an overwhelming urge to light up.

Even if you don't make it the first time, you are not a hopeless case, so don't be discouraged. Simply resolve to start all over again with your decision making, conditioning, and the overcoming of the initial difficulties of withdrawal – always by far the worst part. Remember that, if you can remain an ex-smoker for approximately a month, there is great hope that you will remain an ex-smoker forever. Although you may have to guard against temptation, probably for the rest of your life, the temptations will have diminishing force the longer you go without smoking.

By stopping smoking, you greatly increase the chances of adding several years to your life, and of enjoying better health throughout that longer life. As we have said, all the acute effects of smoking are eliminated within two weeks, and many of the impaired bodily functions will gradually return to normal. Naturally, some effects are permanent and their degree depends upon the number of years you have been a smoker and the amount of cigarettes consumed. But there are other preventive measures open to you to counter-act these influences, such as different eating habits, controlling your blood pressure (if you have a tendency to hypertension), and improving your physical activity and exercise habits. These can compensate for any established damage caused by smoking, while further decreasing your chance of heart and circulatory disease, as well as of lung disease. So, even as a recent non-smoker, you are well on the road to your risk reduction.

Good luck in your effort to break the habit.

20

How to Plan and Perform an Exercise Programme

We have explained why and how lack of physical activity in our automated society on wheels may be a major factor contributing to heart and vascular disease. Indications are that vigorous physical activity, especially on a programmed basis, has multiple beneficial effects on both physical health and emotional balance. Yet relatively few people perform regular exercise after leaving school. It is therefore important, if you are in this category, that you take some precautionary measures before engaging in an exercise programme.

It is likely that at this moment your muscles, your heart, your vascular system, and your lungs are out of condition. It is thus advisable, even if you have no particular symptoms, to see your doctor, and to have a physical examination including an electrocardiogram and chest X-ray, before engaging in any exercise programme vigorous enough to improve your fitness. If you have any limiting factors, your doctor will advise you about the level of physical activity and exercise you may perform without danger. If you receive a clean bill of health, you should start your exercise programme following general rules worked out by many experts in this field.

A particularly good guide has been published by the British Heart Foundation as No. 7 of their Heart Research Series. Entitled *How to Control Your Weight and the Facts about Cholesterol*, it is available from the BHF, 57 Gloucester Place, London W1.

There are three things to consider when starting an exercise programme: first, your age; second, your present weight; and third, your degree and period of past inactivity. With advancing age, you have to be more careful about the level at which you start exercising. Excessive weight requires greater effort to reach a given level of exercise. And, finally, the longer you have been inactive, the less you are able initially to perform certain levels of exercise. Therefore, in

MAXIMUM ATTAINABLE HEART RATE AND TARGET ZONE

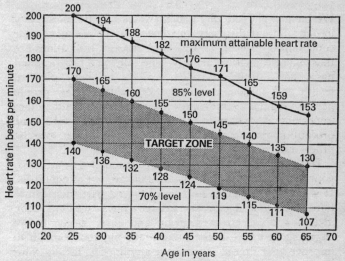

This figure shows that as we grow older the highest heart rate which can be reached during all-out effort falls. These numerical values are 'average' values for age. Note that one third of the population may differ from these values. It is quite possible that a normal 50-year-old man may have a maximum heart rate of 195 or that a 30-year-old man might have a maximum of only 168. The same limitations apply to the 70 per cent and 85 per cent of maximum lines.

Adapted (with author's permission) from Dr Lenore R. Zohman, *Beyond Diet . . . Exercise Your Way to Fitness and Heart Health*, CPC International, Inc. *Source:* Ancel Keys, 'Coronary Heart Disease in Seven Countries', *Circulation*, 41, Supplement I, 1970. Used by permission of the author and the American Heart Association, Inc.

any or all of these cases, you need to start at a comparatively low level and work up gradually to the level necessary to achieve fitness.

I indicated earlier (under 'Exercise and Your Heart') that, to be beneficial, exercise has to reach a target level each time it is performed, and that it also has to be repeated a sufficient number of times. Target levels are most conveniently measured by the heart rate response to given exercises, and the ideal target heart rate is approximately 70

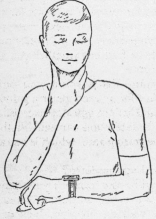

Counting your heart rate.

to 80 per cent of the maximum heart rate an individual can reach, which decreases with age. You can determine your own target heart rate from the chart on page 163.

Do not be over-zealous initially, because if you are unaccustomed to exercise you may experience shortness of breath or fatigue even before you reach your target heart rate. You should stop any time you experience these or any other unusual forms of discomfort. The goal is to work towards reaching your target rate gradually as your muscles adapt, your heart and vascular system become more efficient, and your lungs learn the economy of respiration.

It is easy to determine your heart rate yourself. Simply

count your pulse at rest before you start exercising, then immediately after stopping the exercise at the height of your heart rate, and then again three minutes later. With a little practice, you can find your pulse in several locations, such as over your wrist on the side of your thumb when you press gently down towards the bone, or in your neck an inch below the angle of the jaw. Don't press hard on your neck because you may occlude the blood flow to your brain. Just hold your thumb firmly and gently against the pulsing artery so that you can count the number of pulse beats while looking at your watch. Count the number of beats for ten seconds and multiply by six to get your heart rate per minute. The idea is to count your heart rate only once during each given exercise simply to find out whether you are actually reaching your target rate.

After stopping exercising, immediately count your pulse for *ten seconds only*. Do not count for 15 seconds or a minute because the rate drops very quickly once you stop exercising. When you count three minutes later, you can tell whether your heart has returned to the resting rate, which is its rate before you began to exercise.

What type of exercise should you perform?

The type of exercise that will most improve your physical and cardiovascular fitness is called aerobic or isotonic exercise. This includes brisk walking, jogging, bicycling, swimming, playing tennis, basketball, badminton, squash, and so on. Naturally you should choose the form of exercise that best fits your particular circumstances and life style. I explained earlier that it makes good sense to increase your energy expenditure by using every opportunity to walk and exert your body during the normal activities of the day. This, along with judicious eating habits, will help to maintain your weight within the ideal range. However, such increased everyday exercise alone will at best only minimally improve your physical fitness. To become really fit, you need additional vigorous exercise at least three times a week, not more than two days apart. Experts in the field say that

that amount of exercise, regularly performed, will improve your physical fitness to a desirable level and maintain it there permanently.

To obtain maximum benefit, you must maintain your heart rate near or around your target level for at least 20 to 30 minutes every time you exercise. For most people, some training will be necessary before they become capable of maintaining their target heart rate for this length of time. Depending on the starting level of physical fitness, three to four weeks of regular training are usually sufficient to enable the target to be met. Obviously, you may tailor your exercises to your special needs and circumstances.

Exercises should always start with a warm-up period, then progress gradually, over five to ten minutes, to the attainment of the target heart rate. Once you have maintained your heart rate at this level for the 20- to 30-minute period, you should gradually cool off by walking around slowly, stretching your arms, and taking periodic deep breaths. Don't collapse into a chair or stand immobile. Count your heart rate for ten seconds immediately after stopping your exercise, and then continue your cooling-off period.

As you become practised, you will find that you do not have to count your heart rate every time before and after exercise, because eventually you will be able to estimate very closely whether or not you have reached your target heart rate with the amount of exercise you have performed. Counting the heart rate is only necessary initially, and then occasionally during the exercise programme, to be sure that you are performing the proper amount of exercise.

A good time to exercise is in the morning before breakfast. Another good time is before dinner. However, in both cases rest for 10 to 15 minutes before sitting down to eat. Also do not exercise within two hours after a meal, because a full stomach interferes with the efficiency of your heart at this high level of physical activity.

As you progress in your exercise programme, you will

notice that you are able to reach your target heart rate more easily, and that your stamina increases. If you then want to improve your physical fitness further, you must increase the vigour of your exercise. For instance, if you have initially reached 60 per cent of your maximum heart rate by brisk walking, you may have to change your exercise to jogging or bicycling to reach 70 per cent or, even better, 80 to 85 per cent of your maximum heart rate. You can judge this – and with it your level of physical fitness – by re-evaluating your heart-rate response to a given exercise every three to four weeks.

Once you have attained the level of physical fitness you desire, it is imperative that you continue your regular exercise programme in order to maintain fitness. If for some reason, such as illness, you are not able to exercise for some time – say, a matter of weeks or even months – you must start again at the lower level of your programme and build up gradually. However, once you have reached and stayed at a desirable physical fitness level for a period, and then had to stop, you will reach your previous fitness level faster than the first time – the result of a sort of 'recall' phenomenon by which your muscles and heart and vascular system can be rapidly retrained.

DANGER SIGNS

Even with proper precautions, and a clean bill of health established by physical examination, situations may occur which may worry you while performing your exercise. For example, moving faster up the level of exercise than your condition initially allows may unduly exhaust and discourage you. Muscles aching excessively because they are rusty can have the same effect. These are signs that you should probably start at a lower level and build up more slowly – at a level that your muscles and heart and vascular system can adapt to more gradually. Endurance and tenacity are the key words for success. If you have been totally sedentary and flabby for a long time, you can hardly expect miracles.

Some strange feelings may occur during exercise, especially at the outset, and it is important that you use your judgement to assess their significance. Symptoms which occur several hours after you have exercised are usually less significant than those which occur during or immediately after exercise. However, any feeling of pressure or burning in the centre of your chest, behind your breastbone, during or immediately after exercise, lasting from a few minutes to several minutes, should be reason to contact your doctor, and to discontinue your exercise programme until he has examined you. He may want to do an exercise stress test during which he will record your electrocardiogram to evaluate the nature of the discomfort, and will then advise you whether or not you should continue your exercise programme.

An excellent guideline was published by Dr Lenore Zohman, Director of Cardiopulmonary Rehabilitation at Montefiore Hospital in America, in her booklet about the symptoms you may encounter during exercise, their possible cause, and what to do about them. We reproduce it here with Dr Zohman's and the publisher's permission.

A properly and cautiously performed exercise programme, combined with using every opportunity to increase your day-to-day physical activity, will improve your health, your psychological outlook, your self-esteem, and your appearance. However, you should always follow the rules and avoid excess even in exercise. Initial enthusiam is often very high, which leads to impatience and excess, which is what leads in some cases to discouragement and very occasionally to actual risk. I repeat that careful, *gradual* increase in the amount of exercise you take, and persistent repetition of that exercise, are the key words to success.

Any person who modifies eating habits to a heart-saving form, beats the cigarette-smoking habit, and undertakes an exercise programme does a tremendous amount for his

WARNINGS

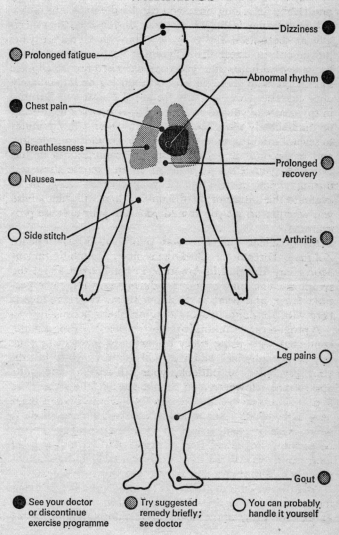

Dizziness

Prolonged fatigue

Abnormal rhythm

Chest pain

Breathlessness

Prolonged recovery

Nausea

Side stitch

Arthritis

Leg pains

Gout

See your doctor or discontinue exercise programme

Try suggested remedy briefly; see doctor

You can probably handle it yourself

WARNINGS AND WHAT TO DO ABOUT THEM*

SYMPTOM	CAUSE	REMEDY
1 Abnormal heart action: e.g. – pulse becoming irregular – fluttering, jumping or palpitations in chest or throat – sudden burst of rapid heart beats – sudden very slow pulse when a moment before it had been on target. (Immediate or delayed)	Extrasystoles (extra heartbeats), dropped heartbeats, or disorders of cardiac rhythm. This may or may not be dangerous and should be checked out by a doctor.	Consult doctor before resuming exercise programme. He may provide medication to eliminate the problem temporarily and allow you to resume your exercise programme safely, or you may have a completely harmless kind of cardiac rhythm disorder.
2 Pain or pressure in the centre of the chest or the arm or throat precipitated by exercise or following exercise. (Immediate or delayed)	Possible heart pain.	Consult doctor before resuming exercise programme.
3 Dizziness, lightheadedness, sudden uncoordination, confusion, cold sweat, glassy stare, pallor, blueness or fainting. (Immediate)	Insufficient blood to the brain.	Do not try to cool down. Stop exercise and lie down with feet elevated, or put head down between legs until symptoms pass. Later consult doctor before next exercise session.

STOP

SEE A DOCTOR BEFORE RESUMING

SYMPTOM	CAUSE	REMEDY
4 Persistent rapid heart action near the target level even 5–10 minutes after the exercise was stopped. (Immediate)	Exercise is probably too vigorous.	Keep heart rate at lower end of target zone or below. Increase the vigour of exercise more slowly. If these measures do not control the excessively high recovery heart rate, consult your doctor.
5 Flare up of arthritic condition or gout, which usually occurs in hips, knees, ankles, or big toe (weight-bearing joints). (Immediate or delayed)	Trauma to joints which are particularly vulnerable.	If you are familiar with how to quieten these flare-ups of your old joint condition, use your usual remedies. Rest and do not resume your exercise programme until the condition subsides. Then resume the exercise at a lower level with protective footwear.
6 Nausea or vomiting after exercise. (Immediate)	Not enough oxygen to the intestine. You are either exercising too vigorously or cooling down too quickly.	Exercise less vigorously and be sure to take a more gradual and longer cool-down.

REMEDIES THAT MAY
BE SELF-ADMINISTERED

SYMPTOM	CAUSE	REMEDY
7 Extreme breathlessness lasting more than 10 minutes after stopping exercise. (Immediate)	Exercise is too taxing to your cardiovascular system or lungs.	Stay at the lower end of your target range. If symptoms persist, do even less than target level. Be sure that while you are exercising you are not too breathless to talk to a companion.
8 Prolonged fatigue even 24 hours later. (Delayed)	Exercise is too vigorous.	Stay at lower end of target range or below. Increase level more gradually.
9 Pain on the front or sides of lower leg. (Delayed)	Inflammation of the fascia connecting the leg bones, or muscle tears where muscles of the lower leg connect to the bones.	Use shoes with thicker soles. Work out on turf which is easier on your legs.
10 Insomnia that was not present prior to the exercise programme. (Delayed)	Exercise is too vigorous.	Stay at lower end of target range or below. Increase intensity of exercise gradually.

CAN BE REMEDIED WITHOUT MEDICAL
CONSULTATION

SYMPTOM	CAUSE	REMEDY
11 Pain in the calf muscles that occurs on heavy exercise but not at rest. (Immediate)	May be due to muscle cramp due to lack of use of these muscles, or exercising on hard surfaces. May also be due to poor circulation to the legs (called claudication).	Use shoes with thicker soles, cool down adequately. Muscle cramp should clear up after a few sessions. If muscle cramp does not subside, circulation is probably faulty. Try another type of exercise, e.g. bicycling instead of jogging, in order to use different muscles.
12 Side stitch (sticking under the ribs while exercising). (Immediate)	Diaphragm spasm. The diaphragm is the large muscle which separates the chest from the abdomen.	Lean forward while sitting, attempting to push the abdominal organs up against the diaphragm.
13 Musclebound feeling in the thigh. (Immediate or delayed)	Muscles are deconditioned and unaccustomed to exercise.	Take hot bath and usual headache remedy. Next exercise should be less strenuous.

* Adapted, with author's permission, from Dr Lenore R. Zohman, *Beyond Diet . . . Exercise Your Way to Fitness and Heart Health*, Mazola Corn Oil, CPC International, Inc., 1974.

CAN BE REMEDIED WITHOUT MEDICAL CONSULTATION

or her heart and vascular system, not to mention his or her general health. But that still leaves all the minor – and sometimes more than minor – aggravations, tensions, and anxieties of daily life. So, let's look at how we might cope better with those in our next chapter.

21

How to Relax

For most people, daily life is filled with tensions, aggravations, and anxieties, and many of them are never going to go away of their own accord. Thus the establishment of a proper rhythm of life requires that we must learn to act decisively when needed to cope with our problems, and then to relax between them in order to recharge our strength and to prepare for our next actions. This conscious engagement and disengagement of the nervous system is really the only way to assure the harmonic function necessary for a well-balanced mental process. However, because so many of us have so many tensions and anxieties, and find it so difficult to achieve the proper cyclic tensing and relaxing of our mental processes, a great many of us have developed the aggressive behavioural pattern known as Type A, a way of behaving that significantly promotes the development of heart disease risk factors. How to relax in these circumstances, and to cope rationally with these problems, is the aim of this chapter.

You have probably already heard about different techniques of relaxation, many of which have been recently imported from Far Eastern countries. There is, for example, yoga, a form of self-discipline and mental relaxation exercise that has its origin in the religious philosophy of Brahminism, which has been widely popularized by modern Western writers. Then there is transcendental meditation, a form of concentration to achieve relaxation and 'cleansing of the spirit'. These and other similar mystical forms of relaxation may well achieve their goal of insight and self-control for some people. However, their mystical or religious trappings make them unattractive to many secular people. Of more appeal to these people may be the scientifically based techniques of relaxation developed by the traditional schools of psychology. These techniques have been applied medically to many thousands of individuals with anxiety and tension, and also used to lower high blood pressure; they are now being practised as group exercises in a number of European countries, especially Germany and Russia, for training workers and others to improve their ability to relax.

All these techniques have the same basic aim of teaching people how to cope with everyday tensions, frustrations, anxieties, and anger, and thus to achieve a balanced emotional state. You too can learn how to relax by training yourself to master the form of concentrative self-relaxation, or autogenic training, that we shall describe here.

The basic concept of the method is not an application of willpower to overcome tension, anger, anxiety, or frustration, because in many cases this simply leads to even more tenseness through a vicious cycle of failure creating even more anxiety, frustration, and anger.

To illustrate what I mean, visualize the father who takes out the frustrations of his job on his children. When they do something wrong or mischievous – even the most minor transgression of the rules in many cases – he explodes and scolds or beats them far beyond any reasonable punishment for the given situation (we see the psychiatric extreme of this in child battering). Most of the time such excessive outbursts are followed by feelings of great remorse and guilt, yet the man cannot prevent further eruptions of his sudden anger and, contrary to all his resolutions to suppress it, is continually faced with his failure to do so. Remorse and guilt are thus magnified by each episode as he attempts to suppress his anger by engaging his willpower; as he attempts to fight a storm with another storm, or fire with another fire.

However, there *is* a solution. Instead of engaging in a

battle between his rising adrenalin and his willpower, such a man could learn to prevent the rise of his uncontrolled emotion and anger in the first place. When he feels the building of tension and the rise of adrenalin, he can prevent the outburst simply by repeating silently to himself, 'I am not angry. I am really not angry. I am relaxed,' until he believes it to be true. Then a simple word of caution or warning to his children would solve the problem.

While this concept of self- or auto-suggestion is described here in very simple terms for the purpose of illustration, it is the principle on which our plan of concentrative relaxation is based. But to make it work you must first understand that relaxing your tensions cannot be achieved by the engagement of your willpower. It is not the engaging of your will that helps you to relax, but the *disengagement* of your willpower and the submission of your entire body and mind to concentrative relaxation.

HOW TO RELAX

The principal aim of concentrative relaxation is to learn how to relax your body by concentrating your mind away from all outside influences and inner disturbing thought processes and on to the simple thought of relaxing. Once you have mastered the technique, you will eventually be able to use it in all situations producing tension, anxiety, and anger, even in the presence of outside disturbances, people, and crowds. At that point you will be able to cope so well with day-to-day fears, anxieties, and anger-making situations that you can decrease your inner tension at any time and in any place.

Acquiring this ability involves learning and practising some particular techniques, which are as follows:

1. You must willingly accept the concept and submit yourself fully to your concentrative relaxation exercise. Negative and sceptical attitudes will lead to failure.

2. Choice of surroundings for the exercise is important initially. You should perform the exercise at first in solitude in your bedroom, or in a room with a bed or couch, that is not too warm and with the light somewhat dimmed. External stimulations such as radio, television, much talk in an adjoining room, or outside street noise should be avoided. You should loosen your clothing so that nothing constricts you.

3. The position of your body is important. For the initial exercise, it is best to lie down on a bed or couch with a pillow under your knees creating a slight bend in your legs. Place your arms next to your body with a slight bend in the elbows (see illustration). Later, you can perform the exercise sitting in an armchair with bent knees and moderately bent elbows, and a rest for your head.

4. Close your eyes, collect your thoughts, and concentrate on your body image and position. This will lead to a certain monotony of happenings in and around you which is necessary for full relaxation.

Arranged thus and lying completely immobile with closed eyes, begin your relaxation exercise by envisioning the words, 'I am completely relaxed', and then repeating them in your mind over and over again. Do not utter a sound or move your lips, but make the entire process a concentration on the meaning of the words as you repeat them internally. Don't open your eyes and don't move any part of your body during this process. By concentrating fully and repeating the words by image fixation on their meaning, sleepiness will not interrupt the exercise. When you have succeeded in concentrating for approximately ten minutes, suddenly terminate the experiment, open your eyes, sit up, and go about your business.

Repeat this exercise once or twice daily for a few days until you feel you have learned to concentrate your thoughts fully on the words, 'I am completely relaxed.' At this point you are ready to start the next task, the cultivation of a feeling of heaviness.

Start out just as before by repeating, 'I am completely relaxed.' Then, when you feel that you have succeeded in maintaining your concentration for two to three minutes on the relaxation words, switch your concentration to the words, 'My arms are very heavy.' Now repeat those words in your mind while imagining your arms lying beside you immobile and very heavy, as if you are unable to move them. This becomes even easier and more successful for many people when they single out one arm only, saying, for example, 'My right arm is very heavy.' It is important not to move your arms in any way, the feeling of heaviness having to be generated in the mind by means of mental concentration only. Continue to repeat and form the mental image, 'My arms are (or my right arm is) very heavy.' After a period of approximately ten minutes of continued concentration, terminate the heaviness task as before by suddenly sitting up and going about your normal activities.

Again, repeat this task once or twice a day, depending on the availability of time and opportunities to arrange the necessary atmosphere. Depending on how well you are eventually able to maintain continuous concentration, you will soon feel a sensation of true heaviness, particularly in your arm, and also in the rest of your body. Ultimately the heaviness can reach the point where you feel you would be unable to move your arm even if you wanted to so long as you continue to concentrate. Once you stop concentrating, of course, you lose both the feelings of heaviness and your inability to move. Two to three weeks of practice are usually necessary to achieve the heaviness feeling within a few minutes of starting to concentrate on it.

Sometimes you may have difficulty concentrating continuously, or even lying still in order to start relaxing, especially in the initial phase when excessive excitement or tension may make the exercise difficult. You may even become restless to the point where you terminate the exercise. Don't let this discourage you. Simply try again later on that day or the next day, continuing a little longer your

concentration on the words, 'I am completely relaxed.'
When you feel that you are able to shut out disturbing
thoughts to the point where you can continuously concentrate on relaxation, switch again to the second task: 'My
arms are very heavy,' or 'My right arm is very heavy.'

While people differ in their capacity for autosuggestion,
almost everybody can learn this relaxation technique by
repeated trial and with sufficient persistence. It should
perhaps be added that the feelings of arm and body heaviness produced by this technique result in objective muscle
relaxation which can be proved by certain measurements of
muscle tension.

It is very important that all details of the entire concentrative relaxation exercise be exactly followed. The prerequisites of solitude, of the described body position, and
of complete submission of all thought processes to the mental concentration must be present. The return to action
after termination of the exercise should also be exactly followed, including a quick opening of the eyes, tensing of the
muscles when sitting up, and then taking several deep
breaths. Submission to concentration, retreat from concentration, and return to normal mental processes should be
decisive actions, so be sure to follow the rules to the letter.

After you can achieve the sensation of heaviness, you
may proceed to the next task, which is the creation of a
feeling of warmth.

You have probably already noticed that when you
achieved complete heaviness in one or both of your arms,
you also experienced a certain feeling of warmth there.
The next step is to concentrate on this warm feeling. Always start by concentrating initially on, 'I am completely
relaxed,' then, when you are able after several weeks of
exercise to reach the heavy feeling quite quickly, switch
your concentration to the thought of warmth by saying to
yourself now: 'My right arm is very heavy and very warm,'
'My right arm is warm.'

The mental image of warmth in the right arm, achieved

by your concentration upon and repetition of the words, will eventually lead to a feeling of warmth, in addition to your feeling of heaviness and immobility. Practise achieving this repeatedly the way you practised the heaviness task. Again, close each session by decisively stopping concentrating, opening your eyes, tensing your muscles, taking several deep breaths, and then getting up and walking away. Practise once a day at least four to five times a week and you should be able to master all three tasks in one or two months.

During your practice of these different tasks, you will begin to notice that the sense of relaxation extends to your entire body, and that the heaviness feeling in your right arm will also, to some degree, be extended to your other extremities. After you have mastered achieving the sensation in one arm, you can and should alternate by concentrating in exactly the same way on both arms, or on both legs, or on all four extremities. The same applies to the warmth sensation. Always start your relaxation, however, with the first task, which is to concentrate on the words, 'I am completely relaxed,' before switching to the feelings first of heaviness and then of warmth. The relaxatory value of a subjective feeling of warmth can also be objectively demonstrated by measuring the skin temperature before and during performance of the task.

During the different degrees of relaxation produced by mastering these techniques, changes in other autonomic body functions can also be observed. Your heart rate will become slower and your heart action will be quieter. Your breathing rate will also decrease because of your resting state and decreased metabolism. Advanced stages of concentrative relaxation can include deliberately quietening the heart action and slowing the heart rate, as well as slowing the breathing. However, such tasks should be supervised by a trained psychologist or doctor.

Once you have mastered the three stages of concentrative relaxation in the lying-down position, you may try to

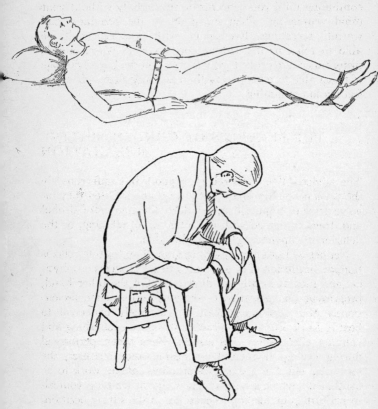

Positions for relaxation exercise, lying down and sitting.

duplicate it in a sitting position in an armchair. You can also do the exercises sitting on an upright chair by spreading your legs somewhat apart, leaning forward, placing your elbows on the centre of your thighs, pointing your hands towards the midline, and hanging your head loosely down (see illustration). After closing your eyes, start as always by concentration on the thought, 'I am completely relaxed,' continuing until you concentrate successfully without your mind wandering. Then move on to the heaviness and warmth sensations. Eventually, with practice, you'll be able to relax in this sitting position even when outside disturbances are present, which gives you the big advantage of being able to relax at any time and anywhere when you feel tension mounting.

THE BENEFITS OF CONCENTRATIVE RELAXATION

The advice, 'You must relax', is good, but unfortunately the ways people do so are not always good. Often they involve drink or tranquillizers – indeed, the amount of alcohol and drugs consumed with the intention of relaxing, or the delusion of 'unwinding', is unbelievable.

Neither will produce anything more than fleeting relaxation, or an illusion of it, and very often the effects on physical and mental health are disastrous. On the other hand, progressive concentrative relaxation, performed conscientiously and persistently, can be extremely beneficial to health. Most people who practise it report a refreshing and calming effect after each session. Even when performed during feelings of mental exhaustion and tenseness, the refreshing effect of a short session often enables work to be continued – which is a great advantage of training yourself to perform your relaxation exercises in the sitting position.

Mastering concentrative relaxation will also enable you to overcome excessive and unnecessary tensions caused by aggravation or other problems when you feel the need of a clear and decisive mind. Indeed, anxieties of different kinds can be overcome by successful relaxation exercises. For example, if you have a groundless fear that you might have a specific illness such as heart disease, or an ulcer, or a mental problem – made groundless by medical examination – relaxation exercises can help you greatly to overcome those anxieties.

Your relaxation exercises can also help you to achieve more restful sleep, or help you fall asleep without a pill when you have difficulty doing so. In this case, do not tense your muscles and get up after termination of the exercise, but just open your eyes for a moment, take a few deep breaths, and say, 'Now I am going to sleep.' Many times this will be more helpful than any sleeping drug.

Concentrative relaxation can also help to lower your blood pressure if you have a tendency to hypertension, by supplementing other interventions, such as weight reduction and medication.

Finally, relaxation exercises can help you to stop smoking, if you are a smoker, by helping you to overcome nervous irritability and tension during the early phases of the giving-up period.

22

How to Live Enjoyably
after a Heart Attack

Medical and technological progress is ever improving the
chances of surviving a heart attack, and there are currently
many millions of living victims of this trauma. If you are one,
you will have been told that it is still not too late to take
care of your heart by the practice of prevention. The tragedy is that it took a heart attack to make you aware of
this.

Blood cholesterol levels, weight, cigarette smoking,
blood pressure, and physical exercise are just as significant
after a heart attack as before it. The risk factors continue
to operate: increased blood cholesterol may plug up new
arteries; continued cigarette smoking will further damage
an already damaged heart; high blood pressure contributes
to the progression of atherosclerosis. All encourage further
heart attacks.

On the other hand, many heart attack victims who now
religiously follow a heart-saver regime, and are regularly
seen by their doctors, enjoy a productive life in relatively
good health. The good news for those who closely follow
such programmes is that progression of their atherosclerosis
can be arrested. I myself have seen many patients, as have
other heart specialists, who show no progression in the
disease upon repeat examination of the coronary arteries
by angiography several years apart. But they are almost
without fail individuals who follow a strict preventive
programme.

Many victims of coronary heart disease who develop
angina, and show partially obstructed coronary arteries by
angiography, can now be helped by surgical bypass of the

blockage, using a piece of vein removed from the leg as a graft. This has resulted in marked health improvement, loss of chest pain, and a relatively normal life. Surgical bypass may even help after a heart attack if chest pain continues and angiography shows more partially blocked coronary arteries, in addition to that which was completely occluded at the time of the heart attack. The partially blocked artery can be surgically bypassed and the chest pain will improve.

However, a very strong warning is needed to prevent any feelings of complacency and false security after restoration of health by surgical bypass of the coronary arteries. A religiously observed preventive programme is still essential, because the same rules apply for progression or development of new atherosclerotic obstructions in the coronary arteries as before. Risk reduction measures are always necessary to prevent new problems from arising.

There are now hundreds of thousands of people who have not yet suffered a heart attack but who have developed a sufficient degree of obstruction in their coronary arteries to produce symptoms of chest pain and have undergone bypass surgery to restore the blood supply to their heart. These individuals are often restored to complete health and normal heart functioning, since no serious damage has yet occurred. However, the same applies to them regarding risk reduction as to the survivor of an actual heart attack. In short, their future depends to a great extent on how closely they follow their heart-saver regimen.

The amount of physical activity, exercise, and work you may perform after recovery from a heart attack, or from coronary bypass surgery, will depend on the amount of damage to your heart muscle and the degree of recovery you have reached. Your doctor, in consultation with a cardiologist, will determine what you can safely do in all these fields. Even after a heart attack a carefully programmed exercise and physical activity regimen is usually beneficial because it improves blood circulation to the healthy, unaffected heart muscle – quite apart from improving a person's feeling of well-being and psychological outlook. However, regular check-ups and proper supervision regarding the amount of exercise you perform are always advisable. There are centres at hospitals throughout the country which have units which specialize in rehabilitation programmes for individuals who have suffered heart attacks or have diagnosed coronary heart disease.

From the foregoing, you can see that the chances for a happy, productive, and extended life have increased tremendously for heart attack and coronary heart disease victims in the past ten years. There is thus every reason to be optimistic and to put aside despair. You can do a lot to improve the quality of your life, and to prolong it. Medical science has advanced beyond most doctors' wildest expectations in the restoration of the health and the function of the ailing heart, and should soon enable us to rescue the dying heart muscle during the early phases of a heart attack, thus preventing further damage.

Medical science, however, has not yet discovered the pill which will dissolve the blockage in your arteries that caused the atherosclerosis, or prevent the development of more atherosclerotic plaques if you ignore all preventive measures. So it is still up to you to do your critical share in this battle.

Endpiece

We have fully examined together in this book the causes, treatment, and prevention of heart and vascular disease. We have shown how the way people live, eat, and generally behave relates to the frequency and causes of heart disease. We concluded that atherosclerosis is the most frequent single cause of heart attacks, strokes, and vascular illness in the civilized Western world, causing over half of all deaths and disability from heart and circulatory disease. We have identified as the major risk factors in the development of atherosclerosis elevated blood cholesterol, high blood pressure, cigarette smoking, and physical inactivity, and we have made it plain that these are the only factors that the individual can do something about. We have shown that by reducing these risk factors, almost everyone can prevent the development and progression of atherosclerosis and thus of heart attacks, strokes, and vascular illnesses.

We have then journeyed with you through your personal life, your environment and its effects on you, your emotional life, and your habits generally. By this point, I believe, you will have decided not to remain a victim of ignorance and inaction. By now you have made, I hope, the decision at least to modify your risk factors, and at best to change them to factors of no risk at all. Obviously, a healthy life without fear of a heart attack or stroke is worth such a decision and the personal effort it involves, because what are wealth and 'success' without the good health to enjoy them?

Medical science has greatly increased your chance of maintaining fine health and full recovery from most illnesses. But the final message is that you still have to do your part: the serum of eternal youth and the magic pill that will cure all ills are still very far away from reality.

And, oh yes, I almost forgot. There are three more things that will help you to lead a healthy and happy life. They are a little faith, a little humour, and a twinkle in your eye.

Glossary

ADRENALIN Secretion of the adrenal gland located above the kidney. It constricts the blood vessels, increases heart rate, and raises blood pressure.

AEROBIC EXERCISE Also called 'isotonic'. It occurs when the muscles involved sustain their oxygen supply during the entire period of exercise.

ALDOSTERONE Hormone secreted by the outer region of the adrenal gland. Released into the blood stream, it makes cells retain sodium (salt) and water to prevent excessive water loss.

ALVEOLI Small air sacs at the end-bronchioles (small air-tubes) in the lung. The exchange of oxygen and carbon dioxide between the blood and inspired air takes place in the alveoli.

ANEURYSM Bulging of the wall of an artery or vein resulting from weakening of the wall.

ANGINA (PECTORIS) Chest pain, often radiating to the left arm and left shoulder, caused by insufficient blood supply to the heart muscle.

ANGIOGRAPHY An X-ray procedure with the use of an opaque material injected into the blood to visualize blood vessels and the heart.

ANGIOTENSIN Constrictor agent of the blood vessels produced by an enzyme released by the kidney (renin) acting on a protein precursor produced by the liver (angiotensinogen).

AORTA The main artery into which the left heart chamber delivers the blood.

AORTIC VALVE Tissue-paper-like structure between the left pumping chamber and the aorta that allows the blood to pass through and closes to backflow when the left pumping chamber relaxes.

ARTERIOSCLEROSIS General term for hardening of the arteries. Could mean stiffening of the arterial wall with or without obstruction of blood flow.

ARTERY Blood vessel that carries oxygen-rich blood from the heart to various parts of the body.

ATHEROSCLEROSIS Deposit of fatty material in the inner wall of an artery, narrowing its passage and inhibiting blood flow.

ATRIOVENTRICULAR (A-V) NODE Small bundle of special muscle fibres between the walls of the two upper chambers of the heart. Electrical impulses controlling the rhythm of the heart are conducted through this muscle bundle from the right upper chamber to the lower chambers.

ATRIUM Receiving chamber of the heart where blood collects after return from organs and lung respectively.

AUTONOMIC NERVOUS SYSTEM Also called vegetative or involuntary nervous system. Controls tissues, glands, smooth muscles, and the heart, which are not under voluntary control.

BENZ-O-PYRENE Strong cancer-producing chemical present in certain tar products and also in cigarette smoke.

BLOOD VOLUME The amount of blood that fills the heart and the blood vessel system.

BRONCHIOLES Small air ducts connecting the larger ducts (bronchi) with the air sacs (alveoli) of the lung.

BRONCHOSCOPY Examination of the air ducts (bronchi) in the lung by introducing a tube containing a mirror.

CALORIES Units of energy obtained from food. One unit is the amount of heat required to raise the temperature of 1 kilogram of water 1 degree centigrade.

CAPILLARY VESSELS Smallest microscopic blood vessels.

CARBON DIOXIDE End product of organic metabolism exhaled into the air, and of burning of organic material.

CARBON MONOXIDE Product of incomplete burning of organic material in the presence of insufficient oxygen.

CARDIAC OUTPUT The amount of blood ejected by the heart in any one minute of time.

CEREBROVASCULAR INSUFFICIENCY Insufficient blood flow to one or more arteries of the brain due to obstruction.

CHOLESTEROL Fat-like substance found in animal tissues and blood.

COAGULATION Process of clot formation.

COLLATERAL CIRCULATION Connection that develops between neighbouring arteries when one of them is partially obstructed.

CORONARY ARTERIES Blood vessels that supply the heart itself. They arise from the aorta in two places across each other just above the aortic valve.

CORONARY SINUS Large vein of the heart that collects returned blood from heart muscle.

DIASTOLE Relaxation phase during each heart beat.

DIASTOLIC BLOOD PRESSURE Pressure in the arteries during relaxation of the heart.

ELECTROCARDIOGRAM Graphic record of the electric currents produced by the heart.

ELECTROPHORESIS Separation of substances by their electric charge in an electric field.

EMPHYSEMA Enlargement of air sacs (alveoli) and destruction of separating tissue between air sacs in the lungs due to obstruction of air ducts (bronchioles), often as a result of cigarette smoking.

EPIDEMIOLOGIST Scientist studying factors which determine the frequency and distribution of a disease in a human community or population.

ESSENTIAL AMINO ACID Breakdown product of proteins (through digestion) necessary for normal bodily functions.

FATTY STREAKS Early deposits of cholesterol in arteries that have not yet produced obstruction. These are visible only at autopsy.

GENES Coding substance in specific parts (chromosomes) of the cell nucleus that determine hereditary traits.

GLUCOSE TOLERANCE TEST Measuring the response of the sugar metabolism to a given sugar load (ingestion of sugarwater) during a period of time.

GROWTH HORMONE Hormone produced by the pituitary gland governing normal growth and having a role in protein metabolism.

HAEMOGLOBIN Iron-containing protein molecule of the red blood cells capable of binding and releasing oxygen and carbon dioxide.

HEART FAILURE Failure of the heart to pump properly, leading to congestion of blood in the lung vessels and other parts of the body (liver, legs, etc.).

HEART MUSCLE DISEASE Weakness of the heart muscle due to inflammation or metabolic disorder of the muscle that leads to heart failure. Also called 'myocardiopathy'.

HYPERTENSION Also called high blood pressure. Increased pressure in the arterial system generated by increased work of the heart against a higher than normal resistance in the small blood vessels.

HYPOCHONDRIA Excessive fear of disease arising

from misinterpreting or imagining symptoms without foundation.

HYPOTHYROIDISM Low thyroid function leading to decreased total body metabolism.

HYPOXIA Oxygen lack of body tissues due to low blood oxygen level or impaired blood circulation.

INTERCOSTAL NEURALGIA Chest wall discomfort due to irritation or inflammation of nerve innervating muscles between two adjacent ribs.

ISOMETRIC EXERCISE Form of exercise that tenses the muscle but does not increase its blood flow.

ISOTONIC EXERCISE See Aerobic Exercise.

KIDNEY DIALYSIS Elimination of waste products, mostly urea, from the blood by passing the blood of an individual through a membrane system called a dialyzer when the kidneys are unable to do so. Usually the blood is taken from an artery of the arm and returned to a vein after passing through a membrane.

LIPOPROTEIN Fat and protein molecules combined as they are carried in the blood circulation.

LYMPH VESSELS Small vessels that carry lymph, a more or less clear to slightly milky fluid, from the gut and other organs to larger veins, passing it through lymph nodes, which act as filters.

MALIGNANT HYPERTENSION Severe hypertension that leads usually rapidly to vascular damage and kidney or heart failure.

MAXIMAL AEROBIC CAPACITY OR POWER The maximum amount of oxygen that can be delivered to the tissues during heavy exercise. It is limited by the amount of blood the heart can deliver (maximal cardiac output).

MAXIMUM HEART RATE The highest heart rate that can be reached with heavy exercise.

MAXIMUM OXYGEN UPTAKE The maximum amount of oxygen an individual can extract from inspired air during heavy exercise. It determines the amount of oxygen that can be delivered to the tissues (maximal aerobic capacity) and is limited by the amount of blood passing through the lungs (maximal cardiac output).

MITRAL VALVE The valve between the left receiving chamber (atrium) and pumping chamber (ventricle) of the heart. This valve has two fine tissue-like leaflets.

MYOCARDIAL INFARCTION Injury and death of heart muscle cells to which the blood supply has been cut off usually by blockage of their supplying coronary artery. The resulting clinical picture is the 'heart attack'.

MYOCARDIOPATHY See Heart Muscle Disease.

NEPHROSCLEROSIS Hardening and narrowing of the small arteries of the kidney as a result of severe hypertension. It leads to kidney disease.

OBSTRUCTIVE LUNG DISEASE, CHRONIC See Emphysema.

OESTROGEN Female sex hormone, produced by the ovaries.

PACEMAKER Small mass of specialized cells in the right receiving chamber (atrium), called sinus node, discharging electric impulses that result in the sequential contraction of the heart known as heart beat. In case of damage and failure of the natural pacemaker, artificial electric pacemakers can be inserted into the heart.

PAPILLARY MUSCLES Muscle bundles in the ventricle protruding towards the inside of the chamber. At their free edge, they are attached to thin cords that are anchored to valve cusps.

PITUITARY GLAND A small gland attached to the bottom part of the brain that produces stimulating hormones for other glands so that they maintain their proper hormone production depending on the needs of the body. It produces stimulating hormones for the thyroid gland, adrenal gland, ovaries, etc.

PSYCHOSOMATIC HEART DISEASE Belief by patient that he/she has heart disease based on misinterpretation of discussion, action, or manner of the doctor or his colleagues.

PULMONARY ARTERY The large artery to which the right ventricle of the heart ejects the oxygen-low blood to be distributed and enriched by oxygen in the lung.

RHEUMATIC FEVER Disease sometimes following a streptococcal infection, usually in children. Symptoms may include: fever, swelling of joints, rash, muscle twitching (St Vitus Dance or chorea). The heart may be involved, resulting in scarring of valves, heart enlargement, and other damage.

SEPTUM Connective tissue membrane and muscular dividing wall between the left and right atria and ventricles respectively, separating them completely so that no direct exchange of blood takes place between the two sides.

SEX CHROMOSOMES Particles of cell nucleus carrying the genes that determine sex characteristics of off-spring.

SEX HORMONES Hormones produced by ovaries of females and testicles of males, which regulate sexual functions.

SINUS NODE See Pacemaker.

STREP THROAT Infection of the throat by the bacterium streptococcus. It is characterized by fever, difficulty and pain when swallowing, and white patches on the red, swollen tonsils.

STREPTOCOCCUS, BETA HAEMOLYTIC Bacterium responsible for strep throat, which can result in rheumatic fever.

STROKE Also called cerebrovascular accident or apoplectic stroke. Among the causes are blood clot formation in an artery of the brain, rupture of artery, blood clot carried from the heart to the brain, or tumour of the brain.

STROKE VOLUME   Amount of blood the heart ejects with each contraction.

SYSTOLIC BLOOD PRESSURE   Peak pressure in the artery during contraction of the heart and ejection of blood.

TARGET HEART RATE   Heart rate that should be maintained for a given period of time during exercise for the exercise to result eventually in increased physical fitness. This is usually between 70 and 85 per cent of maximum heart rate.

TREADMILL EXERCISE OR STRESS TEST   A specified amount of brisk walking on a moving platform, level or on an incline, with electrocardiographic leads attached to monitor response of the heart.

TRIGLYCERIDES   Chemical bonds between a glycerine molecule and different fatty acid molecules, the usual form of fats in the blood and in nature.

VEINS   Blood vessels collecting unoxygenated blood from various parts of the body and returning it to the heart.

VENTRICLES   The pumping chambers of the heart. The right ventricle pumps blood to the lungs through the pulmonary artery, the left to various organs through the aorta.

VENTRICULAR FIBRILLATION   Rapid irregular twitchlike contraction of the muscle of the ventricles that renders them ineffective in ejecting blood and maintaining blood circulation. When circulation is not assisted by other means or fibrillation not converted within three to four minutes, the organism dies. The cause of ventricular fibrillation is usually insufficient blood or oxygen supply to an area of the heart such as occurs with myocardial infarction.

Appendix I

Tables of Ideal Weight, Recommended Daily Calorie Intake, and Calorie Equivalents of Exercise for Planning of Weight Reduction Programme.

I. SUGGESTED WEIGHTS FOR MEN BY HEIGHT AND BODY FRAME†

Height ins. (cm)	Small frame lb (kg)	Average frame lb (kg)	Large frame lb (kg)
60 (152)	106 (48)	117 (53)	130 (59)
61 (155)	110 (50)	121 (55)	133 (60)
62 (157)	114 (52)	125 (57)	137 (62)
63 (160)	118 (54)	129 (59)	141 (64)
64 (163)	122 (55)	133 (60)	145 (66)
65 (165)	126 (57)	137 (62)	149 (68)
66 (168)	130 (59)	142 (64)	155 (70)
67 (170)	134 (61)	147 (67)	161 (73)
68 (173)	139 (63)	151 (69)	166 (75)
69 (175)	143 (65)	155 (70)	170 (77)
70 (178)	147 (67)	159 (72)	174 (79)
71 (180)	150 (68)	163 (74)	178 (81)
72 (183)	154 (70)	167 (76)	183 (83)
73 (185)	158 (72)	171 (78)	188 (85)
74 (188)	162 (74)	175 (79)	192 (87)
75 (191)	165 (75)	178 (81)	195 (89)
76 (193)‡	168 (76)	181 (82)	198 (90)
77 (196)‡	172 (78)	185 (84)	202 (92)
78 (198)‡	175 (80)	188 (86)	205 (93)

* Adapted from Frank Konishi, *Exercise Equivalents of Foods: A Practical Guide for the Overweight*, copyright © 1973 by Southern Illinois University Press. Reprinted by permission of Southern Illinois University Press.

† Without shoes and other clothing. Adapted from M. L. Hathaway and E. D. Foard, *Heights and Weights of Adults in the United States*, Home Economics Research Report No. 10, U.S. Department of Agriculture, Washington, D.C., 1960.

‡ Extrapolated values.

2. SUGGESTED WEIGHTS FOR WOMEN BY HEIGHT AND BODY FRAME*

Height ins. (cm)	Small frame lb (kg)	Average frame lb (kg)	Large frame lb (kg)
58 (147)†	94 (43)	102 (46)	110 (50)
59 (150)†	97 (44)	105 (48)	114 (52)
60 (152)	100 (45)	109 (49)	118 (54)
61 (155)	104 (47)	112 (51)	121 (55)
62 (157)	107 (49)	115 (52)	125 (57)
63 (160)	110 (50)	118 (54)	128 (58)
64 (163)	113 (51)	122 (55)	132 (60)
65 (165)	116 (53)	125 (57)	135 (61)
66 (168)	120 (54)	129 (59)	139 (63)
67 (170)	123 (56)	132 (60)	142 (64)
68 (173)	126 (57)	136 (62)	146 (66)
69 (175)	130 (59)	140 (64)	151 (69)
70 (178)	133 (60)	144 (65)	156 (71)
71 (180)	137 (62)	148 (67)	161 (73)
72 (183)	141 (64)	152 (69)	166 (75)
73 (185)	145 (66)	156 (71)	171 (78)
74 (188)	149 (68)	160 (73)	176 (80)
75 (191)	153 (69)	164 (74)	181 (82)

* Without shoes and other clothing. Adapted from Hathaway and Foard.

† Extrapolated values.

3. RECOMMENDED CALORIES PER DAY FOR MEN BY WEIGHT AND AGE*

Body weight lb (kg)	Cal per day Age (in years)				
	22	35	45	55	65
110 (50)	2,200	2,100	2,000	1,950	1,850
120 (54)	2,350	2,250	2,150	2,100	1,950
130 (59)	2,500	2,400	2,300	2,250	2,100
145 (66)	2,650	2,500	2,400	2,350	2,200
155 (70)	2,800	2,650	2,600	2,500	2,400
165 (75)	2,950	2,800	2,700	2,600	2,500
175 (79)	3,050	2,900	2,800	2,700	2,600
190 (86)	3,200	3,050	2,950	2,850	2,700
200 (91)	3,350	3,200	3,100	3,000	2,800
210 (95)	3,500	3,300	3,200	3,100	2,900
220 (100)	3,700	3,500	3,400	3,300	3,100
230 (105)	3,850	3,650	3,550	3,450	3,250
240 (109)	4,000	3,800	3,700	3,600	3,400
250 (114)	4,150	3,950	3,850	3,750	3,550

*Adapted from National Research Council, *Recommended Dietary Allowances*, 7th edn., National Academy of Sciences, Washington, D.C., 1968.

4. RECOMMENDED CALORIES PER DAY FOR WOMEN BY WEIGHT AND AGE*

Body weight	Cal per day Age (in years)				
lb (kg)	22	35	45	55	65
90 (41)	1,550	1,500	1,450	1,400	1,300
100 (45)	1,700	1,600	1,550	1,500	1,450
110 (50)	1,800	1,700	1,650	1,600	1,500
120 (54)	1,950	1,850	1,800	1,750	1,650
130 (59)	2,000	1,900	1,850	1,800	1,700
135 (61)	2,050	1,950	1,900	1,850	1,700
145 (66)	2,200	2,100	2,000	1,950	1,850
155 (70)	2,300	2,200	2,100	2,050	1,950
165 (75)	2,400	2,300	2,200	2,150	2,000
175 (79)	2,500	2,400	2,300	2,200	2,100
185 (84)	2,600	2,500	2,400	2,300	2,200
200 (90)	2,800	2,650	2,600	2,500	2,350

*Adapted from National Research Council, *Recommended Dietary Allowances*.

5. DAYS REQUIRED TO LOSE 5 TO 25 POUNDS BY LOWERING DAILY CALORIE INTAKE

Reduction of calories per day (in kcal)	Days to lose 5 lb	Days to lose 10 lb	Days to lose 15 lb	Days to lose 20 lb	Days to lose 25 lb
100	150	300	450	600	750
200	75	150	225	300	375
300	50	100	150	200	250
400	38	75	114	150	190
500	30	60	90	120	150
600	25	50	75	100	125
700	22	44	66	88	110
800	19	38	57	75	95
900	17	34	51	68	85
1,000	15	30	45	60	75
1,200	11	22	33	44	55
1,500	5	10	15	20	25

6. DAYS REQUIRED TO LOSE 5 TO 25 POUNDS BY WALKING* AND LOWERING DAILY CALORIE INTAKE

Minutes of walking	+	Reduction of calories per day (in kcal)	Days to lose 5 lb	Days to lose 10 lb	Days to lose 15 lb	Days to lose 20 lb	Days to lose 25 lb
30		400	27	54	81	108	135
30		600	20	40	60	80	100
30		800	16	32	48	64	80
30		1,000	13	26	39	52	65
45		400	23	46	69	92	115
45		600	18	36	54	72	90
45		800	14	28	42	56	70
45		1,000	12	24	36	48	60
60		400	21	42	63	84	105
60		600	16	32	48	64	80
60		800	13	26	39	52	65
60		1,000	11	22	33	44	55

* Walking briskly (3.5–4.0 mph), calculated at 5.2 Cal/minute.

7. DAYS REQUIRED TO LOSE 5 TO 25 POUNDS BY BICYCLING* AND LOWERING DAILY CALORIE INTAKE

Minutes of bicycling	+	Reduction of calories per day (in kcal)	Days to lose 5 lb	Days to lose 10 lb	Days to lose 15 lb	Days to lose 20 lb	Days to lose 25 lb
30		400	25	50	75	100	125
30		600	19	38	57	76	95
30		800	17	34	51	68	85
30		1,000	13	26	39	52	65
45		400	22	44	66	88	110
45		600	17	34	51	68	85
45		800	14	28	42	56	70
45		1,000	12	24	36	48	60
60		400	19	38	57	76	95
60		600	15	30	45	60	75
60		800	13	26	39	52	65
60		1,000	11	22	33	44	55

*Bicycling calculated at 6.5 Cal/minute, at approximately 7 mph.

8. DAYS REQUIRED TO LOSE 5 TO 25 POUNDS BY STEPPING* AND LOWERING DAILY CALORIE INTAKE

Minutes of stepping	+	Reduction of calories per day (in kcal)	Days to lose 5 lb	Days to lose 10 lb	Days to lose 15 lb	Days to lose 20 lb	Days to lose 25 lb
30		400	24	48	72	96	120
30		600	18	36	54	72	90
30		800	15	30	45	60	75
30		1,000	12	24	36	48	60
45		400	20	40	60	80	100
45		600	16	32	48	64	80
45		800	13	26	39	52	65
45		1,000	11	22	33	44	55
60		400	18	36	54	72	90
60		600	14	28	42	56	70
60		800	12	24	36	48	60
60		1,000	10	20	30	40	50

* Stepping up and down on a standard 7-inch step at 25 steps/minute, calculated at 7.5 Cal/minute.

9. DAYS REQUIRED TO LOSE 5 TO 25 POUNDS BY SWIMMING* AND LOWERING DAILY CALORIE INTAKE

Minutes of swimming	+	Reduction of calories per day (in kcal)	Days to lose 5 lb	Days to lose 10 lb	Days to lose 15 lb	Days to lose 20 lb	Days to lose 25 lb
30		400	23	46	69	92	115
30		600	18	36	52	72	90
30		800	14	28	42	56	70
30		1,000	12	24	36	48	60
45		400	19	38	57	76	95
45		600	15	30	45	60	75
45		800	13	26	39	52	65
45		1,000	11	22	33	44	55
60		400	16	32	48	64	80
60		600	14	28	42	56	70
60		800	11	22	33	44	55
60		1,000	10	20	30	40	50

* Swimming at about 30 yards/minute calculated at 8.5 Cal/minute.

10. DAYS REQUIRED TO LOSE 5 TO 25 POUNDS BY JOGGING* AND LOWERING DAILY CALORIE INTAKE

Minutes of jogging	+	Reduction of calories per day (in kcal)	Days to lose 5 lb	Days to lose 10 lb	Days to lose 15 lb	Days to lose 20 lb	Days to lose 25 lb
30		400	21	42	63	84	105
30		600	17	34	51	68	85
30		800	14	28	42	56	70
30		1,000	12	24	36	48	60
45		400	18	36	54	72	90
45		600	14	28	42	56	70
45		800	12	24	36	48	60
45		1,000	10	20	30	40	50
60		400	15	30	45	60	75
60		600	12	24	36	48	60
60		800	11	22	33	44	55
60		1,000	9	18	27	36	45

* Jogging – alternate jogging and walking, calculated at 10.0 Cal/minute.

Appendix II

Sample Low-Fat, Low-Cholesterol Menus

MENU NO. 1

BREAKFAST

One half glass (4 oz.) of orange juice
Bran flakes with one half cup of dried skimmed milk
One slice of whole-wheat bread with one
  pat of low-calorie margarine and jam
Two cups of coffee or decaffeinated coffee
  with dried skimmed milk and non-calorific sweetener

Total calories 354
Fats: 10% of total calories

LUNCH

Fish sandwich (haddock, fillet of sole, or the like)
Fresh fruit (not grapes or bananas)
One glass of low-calorie carbonated beverage

Total calories 370
Fats: 20% of total calories

DINNER

Small bowl of consommé
Tossed salad with vinegar and oil
Grilled lean steak, 6 oz.
Baked potato, medium size

Two pats of low-calorie margarine
Small portion of Brussels sprouts
One slice of angel food cake
One cup of coffee or decaffeinated coffee with
  dried skimmed milk and non-calorific sweetener

> *Total calories*   686
> *Fats: 20% of total calories*

> *Total daily calories, 1,410*
> *Fats: 17.5% of total daily calories*

MENU NO. 2

BREAKFAST
One half glass of orange juice
Oatmeal cereal, cooked with 2 oz. of dried
  skimmed milk
One poached egg
One slice of whole-wheat bread with
  one pat of low-calorie margarine
Two cups of coffee with dried skimmed milk or
  non-dairy cream and non-calorific sweetener

> *Total calories*   390
> *Fats: 26.5% of total calories*

LUNCH
Small bowl of vegetable soup
Tuna fish salad with lettuce, tomato
  slices, and crispbreads
One glass of iced tea or iced coffee with
  one-calorific sweetener

> *Total calories*   365
> *Fats: 42% of total calories*

DINNER
One cup of thick soup with two
  savoury biscuits

Webb lettuce with sweet-and-sour dressing
  (made with non-dairy cream)
Grilled fillet of salmon, 6 oz.
One cup of green peas with one pat of
  low-calorie margarine
Baked potato, medium, with one pat of
  low-calorie margarine
One cup water-ice
One cup of coffee or decaffeinated coffee
  with non-dairy cream and non-calorific
  sweetener

Total calories 670
Fats: 12% of total calories

Total daily calories 1,425
Fats: 23.8% of total daily calories

Index

Action on Smoking and Health (ASH), 158

Adenocarcinoma, 153

Adler, Alfred, 98

Adrenal glands, 39, 40–41, 50, 190

Adrenalin, 100, 177, 190

Aerobic capacity, 139, 194, 195

Aerobic exercise, 138, 165, 190

Age:
   relation to heart disease, 63–4, 69, 84–5, 92–3
   sports performance peak, 91

Aggressive behaviour type, 56–7, 100; see also Type A behaviour

Ageing, 80, 91–2, 93

Air pollution, 103–5, 134

Air sacs, lung, see Alveoli

Alcohol consumption, 59, 100, 118–19
   as cause of heart muscle weakness and heart failure, 37

Alcoholism, 37

Aldosterone, 41, 190

Alveoli (air sacs), 24–5, 128, 129, 190, 192

Amino acids, essential, 112, 193

Aneurysm, 97, 190

Angina (pectoris), 30, 46–7, 56, 66, 129, 185–6, 190

diagnosis, 66

Angiography, 185–6, 190

Angiotensin, 71–2, 190

Animal fats, 49, 63, 76, 102, 112–13, 118–19, 144, 145, 146; see also Saturated fats

Aorta, 25, 28, 92, 190
   aneurysm of, 97

Aortic valve, 84, 191

Apoplectic stroke, 196–7

Arteries, 191
   carotid, 71
   collateral, 47, 58, 138
   coronary, 28–30, 31, 46–7, 58, 133, 185–6, 192
   elasticity of, 91–2
   hardening of, 37, 39, 46, 53, 133, 191
   occlusion of, 39
   pulmonary, 24, 196

Arteriosclerosis (hardening of the arteries), 37, 39, 46, 53, 85, 92, 133
   defined, 191

Arthritic chest pain, 65

Atherosclerosis, 31–2, 33, 46, 48–9, 51–6, 70–73, 74–5, 79, 144, 187
   age and, 93
   arrest of, after heart attack, 185–6

Atherosclerosis—*cont.*
of blood vessels of the kidneys, 31, 40–41, 70, 72
as cause of coronary heart disease, 12, 31, 46, 48, 59
as cause of stroke, 39, 70–71, 74, 144, 188
causes and risk factors, 48–53, 76–7, 188
cholesterol, 12, 48, 50–52, 58, 76–7, 104, 113, 114, 119, 133, 137, 143–4, 185, 188
high blood pressure, 52, 149, 185, 188
lipoprotein abnormality, 52, 76
smoking, 53–6, 86, 104–5, 129–34, 188
defined, 31, 48, 191
early signs of, 49
hereditary tendency for, 52, 76
prevention, 74–6, 78, 113–14, 137–8
relationship to psychological makeup, 56–7
sex-related differences, 85–6, 93
susceptibility of Western populations to, 49, 113
treatment, 71–2, 75–6, 77–8, 85–6
vitamins C and E and, 114–15
Atria (collecting chambers), 22–5, 28–9, 191
synchronization with ventricles, 25–7
Atrioventricular (AV) node, 27, 191

Autonomic nervous system, 99, 191
effect of nicotine on, 128
Autoregulation, 30
Autosuggestion, 177–81

Behavioural characteristics, and heart disease, 56–7, 62, 80, 90, 95, 96–7, 99–101, 175
Benz-o-pyrene, 134, 191
Beta haemolytic streptococcus, 33–5, 196
Biofeedback, 80
Blood:
carbon monoxide concentration in, 54–6, 104–5, 133
cholesterol level, 12, 51, 52–3, 56–8, 62–3, 113, 119
viscosity of, effect of smoking on, 55, 133
Blood flow, 19–22
coronary, 29–30, 46–8
resistance to, 38–9, 58, 128
Blood pressure, 29–30, 137
average, 38
diastolic, 29–30, 38, 92, 192
effect of ageing on, 91–3
effect of glomerulonephritis on, 34
effect of nicotine on, 53, 128, 129
effect of salt intake on, 42–3, 44–5, 72, 84, 149–50
and filtration pressure, 51
high, 30, 37, 38–9, 193; *see also* Hypertension
low, 30
during physical activity, 38, 58–9

regulation of, 29–30, 38, 39–41

regulatory malfunction, 40–42, 43–5, 71–2

during sex act, 123

systolic, 29, 38, 46, 92, 197

in Type A vs. Type B people, 56–7

Blood vessels (*see also* Aorta; Arteries; Capillaries; Veins):

artificial, 78, 79

atherosclerotic obstruction of, 31, 40, 47–9, 51–2, 55–6; *see also* Atherosclerosis

congenital defects of, 35–6

dilation and constriction of, 20, 38, 39–40, 41–2, 72

effect of nicotine on, 53–4

effects of ageing on, 91–3

'fatty streaks' in, 49, 51

lining of, 31, 47, 48, 55

resistance to flow in, 38–9, 58

total length of, 20

Blood volume, 40, 44, 191

Body build, 94, 97; *see also* Physique

Brain, 26–7, 30, 31, 37

arterial clotting in, 70–71

arterial rupture in, 70–71

Breathlessness, 56, 66

British Heart Foundation, 45, 162

cookbook of, 148

Heart Research Series, booklet 7 of, 162

Bronchioles, 128, 191, 193

Bronchitis, chronic, 129

Bronchoscopy, 191

Butter, in diet, 145

Bypass grafts, 71, 72, 79, 185–6

Caloric intake, 102, 110, 111–12, 113, 121, 135–7, 144–5, 146, 147–8, 149

Calorie, defined, 192

Cancer, 9, 12, 79, 134, 146, 153; *see also* Lung cancer

Capillaries, 20, 28, 192

Carbohydrates, 110, 111–12, 113–14, 146, 147–8

Carbon dioxide, 20, 24–5, 192

Carbon monoxide, 192

as factor in atherosclerosis, 54–6, 103–4, 129–33

Cardiac arrest, 77

Cardiac output, 19, 25, 38, 44, 192

and aerobic capacity, 139, 194–5

in men vs. women, 83

and oxygen uptake, 195

Carotid artery insufficiency, 71

Central nervous system, 26, 30, 37, 120

and blood pressure regulation, 39–40, 41, 43–4, 45

Cerebrovascular accident, 196; *see also* Stroke

Cerebrovascular insufficiency, 71, 192

Cheese, in diet, 112, 146

Chest pain, 64–6, 69

anginal, 30, 46–7, 56, 64, 66, 185–6

diagnosis, 65–6

other causes, 64–5

Cholesterol, 49–53, 62–3, 76–7, 110, 137, 192

Cholesterol—*cont.*
  in atherosclerotic plaques,
    48, 51
  blood level of, 12, 51, 52–3,
    56, 58, 62, 113, 119
  control of level of:
    by diet, 62–3, 76–7, 113–
      14, 143–8
    by drugs, 76–7
  factor in development of
    atherosclerosis, 12, 48–9,
    50–52, 58, 76, 104–5,
    113, 114, 119, 129–33,
    137, 144, 185, 188
  functions of, 50
  metabolism of, 49–51, 76, 89,
    114, 119,
  and obesity, 50, 68, 113
  as risk factor in heart disease,
    50–52, 58, 62, 67–8,
    143–4, 148, 185, 188
  smoking and, 54, 55, 133
  in Type A vs. Type B people,
    56–7
  Vitamin C and, 114
Chronic bronchitis, 129
Circulatory system, 19–22, 23–
  5, 70, 126, 137–8
  ageing of, 91–3
Climate, 102–3
Clotting, blood, 31, 70
  in brain artery, 70–71
  in coronary artery, 47
  tendency in heavy smokers,
    55, 133
  tendency reduced by exer-
    cise, 137–8
Coagulation, 192; *see also*
  Clotting, blood
Coffee drinking, 100, 116, 117–
  18, 120, 146, 156–7

Collateral arteries, 47, 58,
  138
Collateral circulation, 47, 58,
  192
Concentrative self-relaxation,
  176–84
Congenital heart disease, 35–6,
  60, 84, 88–9
  causes of, 35–6
  defined, 35
  incidence of, 35
Coronary arteries, 28, 29–30,
  31, 46–7, 58, 133, 185–6,
  192
Coronary blood flow, 29–30,
  46–8, 133
Coronary care unit, 77–8
Coronary heart disease, 31, 46–
  60, 66, 104, 185–6
  age and, 92–3
  causes of, 45–8
    atherosclerosis, 12, 31, 46,
      48–9, 51–6, 59, 85–6
  chest pain as symptom of,
    30, 46–7, 56, 64, 65–6
  collateral circulation as
    remedial mechanism,
    47, 58
  hereditary factors in, 88–90
  high blood cholesterol in re-
    lation to, 12–15, 49–53
  high blood pressure as factor
    in, 38–9, 45, 52
  incidence in various count-
    ries, 9, 12–15, 102–3,
    111
  prevention of, 59–60
    exercise as factor, 57–9,
      106–8
  relationship of psychological
    makeup to, 56–7, 95

saturated fat intake in relation to, 12–15, 49, 50, 52
sex-related differences, 85–6, 93
smoking as risk factor, 52–3, 55–7, 86, 90, 104–5, 117–18, 129–34
surgical bypass, 185–6
Coronary sinus, 28, 192

Deaths:
from cancer, 9, 12
from heart attack, 77, 188
first attack, 9
physical work intensity related to, 57–8
from heart disease:
increase in, 12
as share of all deaths, 9
from other diseases, 9, 12
from vascular disease, 188
as share of all deaths, 9
Diabetes, 36, 52, 67
Diastole, 29, 192
Diastolic pressure, 29–30, 38, 92, 192
Diet, 144–50
balanced, 111–12, 113, 144–7
differences in various climates, 102–3
nutrient requirements, 110–11
Dietary habits, 111–15, 143–5
and cholesterol level, 49, 62–3, 76–7, 113, 114, 143–8
and hypertension, 42–4, 45, 149–50
Dietary restrictions, 79, 113–14

for blood pressure control, 149–50
for cholesterol control, 62–3, 76–7, 113–14, 143–8
Drugs:
anti-cholesterol, 76–7,
heart attack, 77–8
for hypertension, 42, 75

Eating habits, see Dietary habits
Ectomorphism, 96
Effort angina, 46
Eggs, in diet, 112, 145
Elasticity, arterial, 91–2
Electrocardiogram, 27, 65, 168, 192, 197
Electrophoresis, 76, 192
Emotional response, 94, 95, 96, 98–101, 107–8; see also Behavioural characteristics and heart disease
Emphysema, 129, 192–3
Endomorphism, 96
Endothelium, 31, 34
Environment, 88, 95, 96, 97, 102–5
Exercise, 135–40, 162–74
aerobic, 138, 165
beneficial effects of, 58–9, 120–21, 135–6
best forms of, 138–9, 165
blood pressure during, 38, 58
cardiac output per minute during, 19, 20–22, 25, 38, 83, 139
danger signs, 167–8, 169–73
after heart attack, 185, 186–7
isometric, 128, 194
isotonic, 138, 165, 194

Exercise—*cont.*
    maximum heart rate during,
        19, 26, 83, 139, 163–5
    oxygen uptake during, 83,
        139
    as preventive factor, 57–9,
        78, 106–8, 137–8, 186–7
    stroke volume during, 19
    target heart rate, 139–40,
        163–7, 197

Fats, 49, 76–7, 110, 111, 112–14
    animal vs. vegetable, 49, 62–
        3, 102, 112–13, 118–19,
        144, 145–6
    dietary restrictions, 62–3,
        76–7
    metabolism of, 49–50, 52, 54,
        76, 89, 118–19, 129
    saturated vs. unsaturated,
        12–14, 49–50, 52, 112–
        13, 147–8
    storage in body, 50, 136
Fatty streak, 49, 50–51, 193
Fibrillation, ventricular, 197
Filtration pressure, 51
Finland:
    incidence of coronary heart
        disease in, 12, 13, 102
    saturated fat intake in, 14
Fish, in diet, 145
Foods, 79–80, 102, 110–15,
        144–50; *see also* Diet;
        Dietary habits; Dietary
        restrictions
Freud, Sigmund, 98
Friedman, Mayer, 56, 95, 100
Fruits, in diet, 114, 146

Genetic abnormalities, 35–6,
    83–4, 88–9

German measles, 36
Glomerulonephritis, 34
Grain and grain products, in
    diet, 113, 114, 146
Greece, incidence of coronary
    heart disease in, 12, 13,
    102
    saturated fat intake in, 14

Haemoglobin, 24–5, 193
    carbon monoxide affinity of,
        54–5, 104, 133
Hardening of the arteries, 37,
    39, 46–7, 52–3, 129, 133,
    191; *see also* Arterio-
    sclerosis
Heart:
    artificial, 78, 79
    blood supply of, 28–30
    cardiac output (capacity) of,
        19, 25, 38, 44, 83, 139,
        192
    functioning of, 19–22, 24–32
    as a motor, 25–30
    performance in men vs.
        women, 83–4
    as a pump, 19–25, 30–31, 58
    size of, men vs. women, 83
    stroke volume of, 19, 83, 197
    structure of, 22–4
Heart attack, 47–8, 62, 72, 74,
    76–8, 79, 188
    age and, 93
    death rates, 77, 188
        among heavy-work vs.
        light-work labourers,
        57–8
    first, 77
        deaths from, 9
    in men vs. women, 93

nervous tension and, 62, 95, 107–9
preventive measures, 74–6, 137–8
exercise as preventive factor, 57–9, 186–7
recurrence, 76–7, 185
preventive measures, 76, 78, 185–7
rehabilitation programmes, 77–9, 186–7
relationship of psychological makeup to, 56, 95
risk factors, 66–9, 75–6, 108–9, 188
cholesterol, 58, 143–4, 188
high blood pressure, 45, 188
smoking, 53, 108, 129–33, 188
treatment, 63–70, 77–8, 186–7
warning signals, 77
chest pain, 64–6, 69
indigestion, 63–4, 69
obesity, 67, 69
Heartbeat, 19–20, 26; see also Heart rate
regulation of, 25–7
Heart block, 27
Heart chambers, 22–5; see also Atria; Ventricles
Heart disease:
behavioural characteristics and, 56–7, 62, 89–90, 95, 100–101
causes of, 33–60
alcoholism, 37, 59
atherosclerosis, 12, 31–2, 33, 46, 48–9, 51–6, 59, 70–73, 74–5, 79, 144, 187
congenital, 35–6, 59–60; see also Congenital heart disease
metabolic disorders, 36, 37, 52, 59
rheumatic fever, 33–5, 59; see also Rheumatic heart disease
summarized, 59–60
viral infections, 36, 59
coronary, see Coronary heart disease
deaths from, 9, 12, 188
early warning signals, 63–70
in men vs. women, 63, 83–6, 93
prevention and treatment, 60, 74–8; see also Dietary restrictions; Exercise; Preventive action
psychosomatic, 70, 194
relationship of age to, 91–3
risk factors, 66–9, 89–90, 108–9, 188
cholesterol, 48–9, 50–52, 58, 62–3, 67–9, 143–4, 148, 185, 188
heredity, 42, 43, 52, 62, 67, 69, 76, 87–90
high blood pressure, 30, 38–9, 45, 59, 67–8, 69, 185, 188
smoking, 53–6, 67–8, 69, 86, 104–5, 118, 125–6, 128–34, 151, 185, 188
Heart failure, 36–7, 39, 59, 193
Heart muscle, 30, 31
autoregulation of blood flow to, 30
contraction of, 25–7, 29, 46
lack of blood flow to, 46–8

Heart muscle disease, 36–7, 59, 193

Heart rate, 19–20, 58
  determining, 164–5
  effect of nicotine on, 53, 128, 129
  during exercise, 19, 26, 83
  exercise target rate, 139–40, 162–7, 197
  maximum, 19, 26, 83, 163–5, 195
  in men vs. women, 83
  at rest, 19, 26, 83
  during sex act, 123–4
  slowed by concentrative relaxation, 181

Heart surgery, 36, 78

Heart transplants, 16

Heart valves, 22–5; see also Valvular disease
  aortic, 84, 191
  artificial, 78, 79
  damage from scarlet fever, 34
  mitral valve, 84, 195
  rheumatic scarring of, 34, 84

Heat, effect of, 102–3

Heavy metals, and high blood pressure, 43

Height, body, 94–5

Hereditary heart defects, 35

Heredity, as risk factor, 61–2, 67, 69, 87–90, 97
  in atherosclerosis, 52, 76
  in coronary heart disease, 88–90
  in high blood pressure, 42, 43, 87–9

High blood pressure, see Hypertension

Hormones, 20, 196
  blood-pressure raising, 40–42
  cholesterol as chemical base for, 50
  growth, 94, 193
  sex, 83–4, 85–6, 196
  thyroid, 96

Humidity, effect of, 103

Hyperlipidemia, 89

Hypertension (high blood pressure), 30, 38–46, 59, 74–5, 79, 185
  age-related differences in, 84–5
  animal studies with rats, 42, 44
  asymptomatic, 75
  as cause of stroke, 39, 45, 70, 188
  causes of, 38–46
    adrenal tumour, 40–41
    arterial obstruction in kidney, 40–42, 71–2
    hereditary factors, 42, 43, 89
    life-style factors, 42–5
    racial factors, 42
  defined, 30, 193
  drinking water and, 43, 116–17
  essential, 40
  as factor in heart disease, 30, 39, 45, 59–60, 67–9, 188
  incidence in Britain and U.S., 45
  malignant, 72, 85, 194
  nervous tension and, 42, 44, 45
  obesity and, 43, 44, 67, 84–5, 149
  prevention, 74–6
  primary, 40, 41–5

relationship to atherosclerosis, 52, 149, 185, 188
relationship to psychological makeup, 57
renal form of, 40–41, 72, 85
sex-related differences, 83–4
treatment of, 41, 44, 74–5
  drugs, 42, 75
  relaxation, 175–6, 184
  surgery, 41, 75
  various consequences of, 39, 45, 51, 52, 70–71
Hypothyroidism, 36, 52, 194
Hypoxia, 104, 194

Indigestion, as warning signal, 63–4, 69
Infant deaths, 12
Infectious diseases, 78, 103
  deaths from, 12
Intercostal neuralgia, 65, 194
Isometric exercise, 138, 194
Isotonic exercise, 138, 165, 194
Italy, incidence of coronary heart disease in, 12, 13, 102
  saturated fat intake in, 14

Japan:
  body height trend, 94
  incidence of coronary heart disease in, 12, 13, 111
  incidence of hypertension in, 43
  research on high blood pressure, 44
  risk score for heart disease, 67–9
  saturated fat intake in, 14

Japanese-Americans, psychological types and incidence of heart disease, 95

Katz, Louis, 85–6
Kidney dialysis, 72, 194
Kidney disease, 74, 79
  as cause of high cholesterol level and atherosclerosis, 52
  high blood pressure and atherosclerosis as cause of, 39, 70, 71–2
  stones, 114
Kidney failure, 72
Kidneys, 37
  atherosclerosis of vessels of, 40, 70, 71–2
  and high blood pressure, 39–41, 43, 72, 85
  renin production, for blood pressure regulation, 41, 71–2
  streptococcal inflammation (glomerulonephritis), 34–5

Legs, atherosclerosis of, 31, 71
Life expectancy, U.K. males, 13
Life-style factors, 12, 60, 96–7, 100–101; see also Dietary habits; Exercise; Nervous tension
  in high blood pressure, 42–6
Lipoprotein, 52, 76, 129, 194
  abnormalities, 76
Liver, 37, 50, 52, 112

Liver—cont.
   in diet, 145
   triglyceride-clearing function
      of, 50, 54, 129
Lumen, 47
Lung, 24, 126, 128, 129
Lung cancer, 55, 61, 104, 134,
   153
Lymph vessels, 50–51, 194

Malignant hypertension, 72,
   85, 194
Marfan's syndrome, 97
Meat, 112–13, 145
Men:
   heart disease in, compared
      with women, 63–4, 83–
      6, 93
   heart performance of, com-
      pared with women, 83–4
   life expectancy in U.K., 13
   symptoms of heart disease,
      63–4, 69–70
Menopause, 84, 85, 86, 93
Menstruation, 84, 93
Mesomorphism, 96
Metabolic disorders as cause of
      heart disease, 36, 52, 59
Metabolism, 95, 96, 137
Michael Reese Research Insti-
      tute, Chicago, 85
Milk, in diet, 112, 146
Minerals, as nutrients, 110–11,
   114
Mitral valve, 84, 195
Myocardial infarction, 47–8,
   56, 85, 195
Myocardiopathy, 37, 193

Nephrosclerosis, 72, 195

Nervous system, 118; see also
   Autonomic nervous sys-
   tem; Central nervous
   system
Nervous tension, 80, 86, 90, 95,
   98–9, 108–9, 135, 175
   and heart attacks, 62, 95
   and high blood pressure, 42,
      43–5
   overcoming, 175–7, 183–4
New Zealand:
   research on high blood
      pressure, 44
Nicotine, 53–4, 128–9, 129–33

Obesity, 50, 67, 69, 84, 90, 95,
   107, 108, 113–14, 121,
   136, 185
   and cholesterol level, 50, 67,
      113–14
   and hypertension, 43, 44, 67,
      84–5, 149
Oestrogen, 85–6, 93, 195
Open-heart surgery, 78
Oral contraceptives, 84
Overeating, 90, 95, 100, 135–6,
   149
Overweight, see Obesity
Oxygen, 20, 24–5, 137, 138
   displaced by carbon mon-
      oxide in smoking, 54–5,
      104, 133
   supply to heart muscle, 30–
      31, 46
   uptake, 83, 139, 195

Pacemaker, 27, 78, 79, 195; see
   also Sinus node

Papillary muscles, 22, 195
Physical activity, 57–9, 106–8, 135–40; *see also* Exercise
Physique, 87–8
  characteristics of, 94
  and heart disease, 96–7
  types of, 96
'Pinched nerve', 65
Pituitary gland, 50, 94, 196
Plaques, atherosclerotic, 46, 47–9, 53, 55–6, 58–9, 187
  in brain artery, 70
  in coronary arteries, 46–9
  description of, 48–9
  development of, 51
  in kidney blood vessels, 40, 71
  in leg arteries, 71
  location of, 51, 72
Polyunsaturated fats, 147–8
Pregnancy, 36, 59, 88, 89
Preventive action, 10–11, 16, 59, 60, 74–8; *see also* Dietary restrictions; Exercise
  importance of, 79–80
  against recurrence of heart attack, 76, 77–8, 185–7
Primary hypertension, 40, 41–6
Proteins, 52, 76
  and hypertension, 43
  in nutrition, 94, 110, 111–14, 144–5, 147–8
Psychodynamic classifications, 56–7, 62, 80, 90, 95, 100, 175
Psychosomatic illness, 99
  heart disease, 70
Pulmonary artery, 24, 196

Racial factors, in high blood pressure, 42
Red blood cells, 24
  carbon monoxide affinity of, 54–5, 133
Relaxation, 156, 175–84
  concentrative, 175, 176–84
Renin, 41, 71–2, 190
Rest:
  blood pressure at, 38
  cardiac output per minute during, 19, 25, 38–9
  heartbeat during, 19, 26, 83
  stroke volume during, 19, 83
Rheumatic fever, 33–5, 59, 196
  incidence of, 35
  susceptibility to, 34
Rheumatic heart disease, 33–5, 59–60, 103
  cause of, 33
  incidence in men vs. women, 83–4
Risk factors, 66–7, 72, 89–90, 108–9, 188
  assessment of risk score, 66, 75–6
  cigarette smoking, 53–7, 67–9, 86, 90, 104–5, 118, 125–6, 128–9, 133–4, 151, 185, 188
  formula for assessment of, 144–5
  heredity, 42, 43, 52, 61–2, 67, 69, 76, 87–90
  high blood pressure, 29–30, 39, 45, 59, 67–9, 149–50, 185, 188
  high cholesterol level, 48–9, 50–52, 58, 62–3, 67–9, 143–5, 148, 185, 188
  interrelationship, 86, 89–90

Risk factors—*cont.*
  physical inactivity, 57–9, 90,
    162, 188
  psychological makeup, 56–7,
    90, 95, 99–101
  reduction of, as preventive
    measure, 75–6
  in Britain vs. Japan, 67–9
Rosenman, Ray H., 56–7, 95,
  100

Salt intake and retention, effect
    on blood pressure, 42–3,
    44–5, 72, 84, 149–50
Saturated fats, 49, 50, 52, 113
    147–8
  relationship to coronary
    heart disease, 12–15, 50,
    52
Scarlet fever, 34
Septum, 22, 196
Sex hormones, 83–4, 85–6, 196
Sex life, 122–4
Sexes:
  differences in heart disease,
    63–4, 83–6
  differences in heart perfor-
    mance, 83–4
Shellfish, in diet, 145
Sinus, coronary, 28, 192
Sinus node, 25–6, 196; *see also*
    Pacemaker
Sleep, 120–21, 124
Smithwick procedure, 75
Smoking, 56–7, 61, 80, 100–
    101, 104–5, 117–18,
    125–34, 151–4
  how to stop, 154–61, 184
  inner need factors, 126
  physiological effects of, 53–6,
    128–9, 133

physiological withdrawal
    symptoms, 127–8
positive vs. negative affect of,
    127, 155, 157–8
psychological addiction to,
    127–8, 158
reasons for, test, 130–32,
as risk factor in athero-
    sclerosis, 52–6, 86, 104–
    5, 133–4, 188
as risk factor in heart attacks,
    53, 133, 185, 188
as risk factor in heart disease,
    53, 68, 69, 86, 90, 104–5,
    117–18, 126, 129, 133–4,
    151, 188
social need factors, 126
Soft drinks, caffeine-contain-
    ing, 118, 146
Sports performance, age of
    peak of, 91
Stomach acid production:
  coffee consumption and, 118,
    146
  effect of nicotine on,
    128–9
Strep throat, 33–5, 59, 196
Streptococcus, 33–5, 59, 103,
    196
Stress, *see* Nervous tension
Stress test, 168, 197
Stroke(s), 74, 77, 79, 90, 196
  atherosclerosis as cause of,
    39, 70, 74, 144, 188
  high blood pressure as cause
    of, 39, 45, 70, 188
  preventive measures, 74–5
Stroke volume, 19, 197
  in men vs. women, 83
Surgery, 36
  bypass, 71, 72, 79, 185–6

for atherosclerosis, 71–2
for hypertension, 41, 75
open-heart, 78
for renal hypertension, 72
Symptoms, 61–70
   breathlessness, 56, 66
   chest pain, 30, 46–7, 56, 64–6, 69
   of coronary heart disease, 30–31, 46–7, 56
   early warning, 63–6, 77
   indigestion, 63–4, 69
Systole, 29
Systolic pressure, 29, 38, 46, 92, 197

Tar, cigarette, 55, 104, 133–4
Target heart rate, 139–40, 162–7, 197
Tea drinking, 116, 118, 120, 146
Tension, see Nervous tension
Therapy, 60, 74–8
   for atherosclerosis, 71–2, 75–6, 77–8, 85–6
   for heart attack, 63–70, 77–8, 186–7
   for high cholesterol, 62–3, 76–7
   for hypertension, 41, 42, 44, 74–5
Thyroid function, low, 36, 52
Thyroid hormone, 96
Transcendental meditation, 175
Treadmill exercise test, 66, 197
Triglycerides, 50, 54, 119, 137, 197
Type A behaviour, 56–7, 62, 90, 95, 100, 175

Unsaturated fats, 12, 14, 49, 147–8
United States:
   incidence of coronary heart disease in, 12, 13, 102
   saturated fat intake in, 14

Valves, see Heart valves
Valvular disease, chronic, 34, 37
Vascular disease, 188
   deaths from, 9, 12
   high blood cholesterol as factor in, 144, 188
   high blood pressure as factor in, 45, 188
   prevention and treatment, 74–8, 188
Vascular spasm, 47–8
Vasoconstrictors, 39–42 passim, 71–2
Vegetable fats, 49, 63, 102, 145–6
Vegetables, 112, 113–14, 115
Veins, 24, 28, 197
Ventricles (pumping chambers), 22–5, 197
   synchronization with atria, 25–7
Ventricular fibrillation, 197
Veterans Administration Cooperative Research Group, 74
Virus infections, as cause of heart disease, 36–7, 59
Vitamins, 110–11, 114–15

'Walk-through pain', 66
Water:
   body requirements, 116

Water—*cont.*
  drinking, 43, 116–17
  and high blood pressure, 43,
      117
  retention in body, 44, 72, 84
Weight control, 44, 95–6
  diets, 113
Women:
  heart disease in, compared
      with men, 63–4, 83–6,
      93

  heart performance of, com-
      pared with men, 83–4
  housework, 108–9
  symptoms of heart disease,
      63–4, 69–70

Yoga, 175
Yugoslavia:
  incidence of coronary heart
      disease in, 12, 13
  saturated fat intake in, 14